Praise for *Your Bones*

"This is a book filled with wisdom and information written in a style which is easy to understand and put to use. I heartily recommend it to all those who care about maintaining a healthy body."

—Bernie Siegel, MD, Author of *Faith, Hope & Healing* and *365 Prescriptions For The Soul*

"*Your Bones* is a down-to-earth guide to osteoporosis, one of the most common health challenges of modern life. If you are 30 or older, you cannot afford to ignore the wisdom in this book."

—Larry Dossey, MD, Author of *The Science of Premonitions, Healing Words,* and *Reinventing Medicine*

"This superb text explains the causes and solutions of osteoporosis, and its associated problems, comprehensively, clearly and accurately. Despite the complexity of the condition, this is an easy read, with no dumbing down of the content—brilliantly highlighting safe, natural, and effective prevention and treatment strategies. Highly recommended."

—Leon Chaitow, ND, DO, Honorary Fellow,
University of Westminster, London
Editor-in-Chief, *Journal of Bodywork &
Movement Therapies*

"This is one of the best books ever written on bone health—absolutely fantastic! In this book, Lara Pizzorno, MA provides scientifically based advice for men and women of all ages to help them develop and maintain strong healthy bones. She makes a complex issue easily comprehensible and provides information that empowers the reader to take measures towards ensuring their own bone health. I highly recommend it."

—George Mateljan, Philanthropist, Author
of the book, *The World's Healthiest Foods*

Your Bones

Your Bones

*How **You** Can Prevent Osteoporosis
& Have Strong Bones For Life—
Naturally*

Lara Pizzorno, MA, LMT
with Jonathan V. Wright, MD

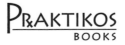

DISCLAIMER

Ideas and information in this book are based upon the experience and training of the author and the scientific information currently available. The suggestions in this book are definitely not meant to be a substitute for careful medical evaluation and treatment by a qualified, licensed health professional. The author and publisher do not recommend changing or adding medication or supplements without consulting your personal physician. They specifically disclaim any liability arising directly or indirectly from the use of this book.

Praktikos Books

P.O. Box 118
Mount Jackson, VA 22842
888.542.9467   info@praktikosbooks.com

Praktikos Books are produced in alliance with Axios Press.

Library of Congress Cataloging-in-Publication Data

    Pizzorno, Lara.
    Your bones : how you can prevent osteoporosis & have strong bones for life naturally / Lara Pizzorno with Jonathan V. Wright.
    p. cm.
    Includes bibliographical references and index.
    ISBN 978-1-60766-007-1 (pbk.)
    1. Osteoporosis—Prevention—Popular works. 2. Osteoporosis—Diet therapy—Popular works. 3. Osteoporosis—Nutritional aspects—Popular works. 4. Osteoporosis—Exercise therapy—Popular works. I. Wright, Jonathan V. II. Title.

RC931.O73P53 2011

616.7'16–dc22

                            2010042333

Contents

PART 2: WHY CONVENTIONAL MEDICINE IS NOT THE ANSWER FOR STRONG BONES

PART 3: WHAT INCREASES YOUR RISK FOR OSTEOPOROSIS?

PART 4: HOW TO HAVE STRONG BONES FOR LIFE

Tables

Preface

WOMEN TODAY ARE REINVENTING WHAT "OLD age" looks like. You *can* have strong bones for life, naturally.

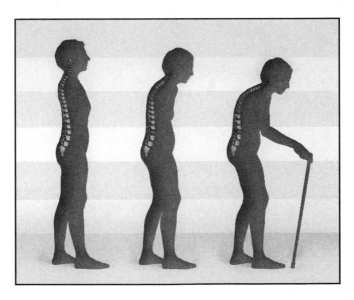

The photo on the back cover is of me, *Your Bones* co-author Lara, aged 60, on a 2009 Mother's Day hike in Stehekin, Washington. I was diagnosed with osteopenia in my very early 50s. Today, I have strong, healthy bones, which I credit to having done everything recommended in this book. I am genetically at very high risk for osteoporosis, but now I will be the first woman in my family in all the generations I know about not to die an osteoporosis-related death. You too can have strong, healthy bones for life.

PART 1

You Are at Risk for Osteoporosis

CHAPTER 1

If You Are a Woman, You're at High Risk for Osteoporosis

What Is Osteoporosis?

OSTEOPOROSIS—LITERALLY, "POROUS BONE" (osteo = bone, porosis = porous)— is a progressive loss of bone that results in bone thinning and increased vulnerability to fracture. Osteoporotic fractures—also called *fragility fractures* because they happen in thinned out, fragile bone—occur primarily in the wrist, rib, spine, and hip, often during daily activities, such as stepping off a curb, which should normally pose no risk for a fracture.[1]

Why Are Women at Higher Risk Than Men of Losing Too Much Bone?

For two key reasons:

First, women start out with less bone than men. Women's peak bone mass is naturally less than men's because women are smaller and have less muscle. When we use our muscles, the muscle contractions put stress on bone, to which it responds by becoming stronger. Men's larger muscles produce stronger contractions, resulting in more stress and approximately 35–40% larger bones.[2]

Secondly, the female hormones, estrogen and progesterone, play vital roles in bone remodeling, and levels of both hormones drop with menopause (medically defined as the last menstrual period); for most women in the Western world, the median age for menopause is 51, but the range for its onset is large—generally between ages 42 and 58. Estrogen prevents excessive action by *osteoclasts*, specialized bone cells that remove worn out or dead bone to make room for new bone. Progesterone is required by *osteoblasts*, the bone-forming cells that pull calcium, magnesium, and phosphorous from the blood to build new bone. Production of both hormones greatly declines during a woman's transition through menopause, resulting in increased bone resorption and decreased formation of new bone.

Am I Really at Risk? How Common Is Osteoporosis?

If you are a woman, the answer is emphatically "Yes!" One in four women will develop osteoporosis after menopause. Lifetime risk for fragility fractures, an indicator of osteoporosis, is 50% in women versus 25% in men.[3] Twenty-five million Americans have osteoporosis or are at significant risk for it.[4] Osteoporosis is responsible for at least 1.5 million fractures each year, including 250,000 hip fractures.

Men Are Not Immune to Osteoporosis

Although women are most at risk, 25–33% of men will experience an osteoporotic fracture in their lifetime. In men, however, the rapid increase in fracture risk begins later, at approximately age 70.[5]

What Are My Chances of Recovering from a Hip Fracture Due to Osteoporosis?

Nearly one-third of all women and one-sixth of all men will suffer an osteoporotic hip fracture. The most catastrophic of fractures, hip fracture leads to death in 12–20% of cases and long-term nursing home care for over 50% of those who survive.

Men fare even worse than women after a hip fracture: a woman's risk of death doubles, a man's risk more than triples.[6] For virtually everyone who suffers an osteoporotic hip fracture, life never returns to "normal."

This is something you definitely want to prevent, and fortunately you can, but *not* by relying on the patent medicines (also called "pharmaceuticals" and/or "drugs") prescribed to prevent osteoporosis.

PART 2

Why Conventional Medicine Is Not the Answer for Strong Bones

The Patent Medicines Prescribed to Prevent Osteoporosis Should Be Your *Last* Choice for Healthy Bones

T'S TRUE, AS SALLY FIELD EMPHASIZES IN HER TV ADS for Boniva®, that you have only one body. It's *not* true that Boniva® or the other bisphosphonate patent medicines commonly prescribed to prevent osteoporosis offer the best way to take care of it!

PATENT MEDICINES

Patent medicines are not a "relic of the past"! They've been with us all our lives. The overwhelming number of prescriptions written in the United States for the entire 20th century and thus far in the 21st century have been for written for patented or formerly patented substances. Even though today's gigantic patent medicine companies try their best to disguise this obvious fact by calling their products "pharmaceuticals," they're still just patent medicines under another name.

All patent medicines have the same basic problem by law: a patent can only be "granted" for substances never, ever found in human bodies or anywhere else on planet Earth. Although it sounds strange, it's literally true to say that patent medicines are "extraterrestrial, space alien" substances!

Since our bodies were designed (or evolved) from entirely natural materials, patent medicines are fundamentally incompatible with design of the human body. It's no wonder more than 100,000 Americans die from patent medications every year, and hundreds of thousands more experience serious adverse effects.[7] By contrast, according to the most recent report of the American Association of Poison Control Centers, not a single American died in 2008 from the use of vitamins, minerals, amino acids, essential fatty acids, hundreds of other supplemental nutrients, or any of thousands of herbal products.[8]

Given this enormous difference in safety, why aren't medical research and medical practice focused on safe and effective natural substances? You've heard of "follow the money"? Here it is again: Because of that patent, no competition is allowed, so patent medicines that cost 98¢ a unit to produce can be (and are) sold for $98 a unit (100 times their cost), or more. Natural substances are also sold at a profit, but competition limits the profit margin to 2 to 3 times cost of production. Predictably, the focus of patent medicine (pharmaceutical) companies is profit, first and foremost. Your health is a secondary goal.

In our opinion, patent medications should always be the last choice for treatment of illness, used only when "body-compatible" natural substances or energies are not available to do the job. Even then, patent medicines should be used with great caution and for the shortest time possible.

The Patent Medicines Prescribed for Osteoporosis, the Bisphosphonates (e.g., Fosamax®, Actonel®, Boniva®, Reclast®), Have Very Nasty Side Effects

Although prescribed to 30 million Americans each year, the bisphosphonate patent medicines (the oral forms, including Fosamax®, Boniva®, Actonel®, and the latest additions to the bisphosphonate arsenal, the once yearly IV-administered patent medicines Reclast® and Aclasta®), are well known to be dangerous.

An FDA alert, issued January 2008, warned physicians that all bisphosphonate patent medicines may cause "severe and sometimes incapacitating bone, joint, and/or muscle (musculoskeletal) pain . . . [which] may occur within days, months, or years" after starting the medication, and in some patients, may not resolve *even after discontinuing the patent medicine.*[9]

Even more alarming, these patent medicines have now been conclusively linked to a number of other serious adverse side effects including *osteonecrosis of the jaw* (jaw bone death, osteo = bone, necrosis = death), *atrial fibrillation* (irregular heartbeat), and increased risk of bone fragility leading to bone fracture—yes, that's right, an *increased risk of bone fracture from the very patent medicines prescribed to prevent it*!

Bisphosphonates Don't Build Healthy, New Bone—They Cause Retention of Old, Brittle Bone

The bisphosphonate patent medicines suppress the activity of *osteoclasts*, the body's specialized cells whose job it is to remove worn out, injured, or otherwise damaged bone. This is a task that must be taken care of before such weakened bone can be replaced with new strong bone.

Osteoclasts are the first phase of the bone renewal process. They take out the bone "trash" to make room for new bone. If osteoclasts are prevented from doing this necessary job—which they very effectively are by bisphosphonates, which work by literally poisoning osteoclasts—damaged bone is left in place rather than cleared out, so no room is made for new bone to be laid down. Eventually, the amount of unhealthy, compromised bone tissue accumulates to the point that bones become very fragile, and any trauma or insult heals poorly, if at all.

The bisphosphonates don't just inhibit, they virtually crush all new bone formation. Researchers at the University of Texas performed bone biopsies on nine women who had been taking Fosamax® for 3 to 8 years, but had nevertheless suffered non-spinal fractures (in the lower back, ribs, hip, or femur) while performing normal daily activities (walking, standing, turning around). New bone formation in these women was nearly *a hundred times lower* than that normally seen in postmenopausal women.[10]

Bisphosphonates Cause Osteonecrosis of the Jaw (ONJ)

In the jaw, bisphosphonates' prevention of normal bone remodeling results in the accumulation of dying bone and its eventual exposure to the inside of the mouth, along with greatly

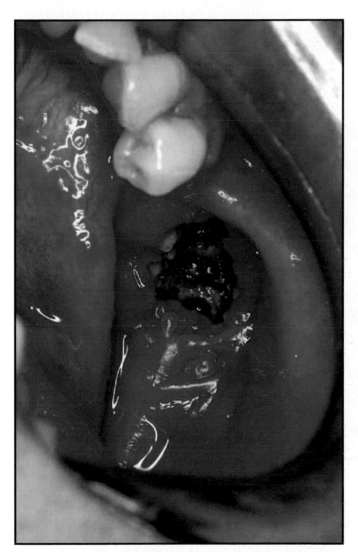

Spontaneous fracture of the lower jaw in woman treated with Aredia® and Zometa® for 24 months (43 years old, breast cancer).

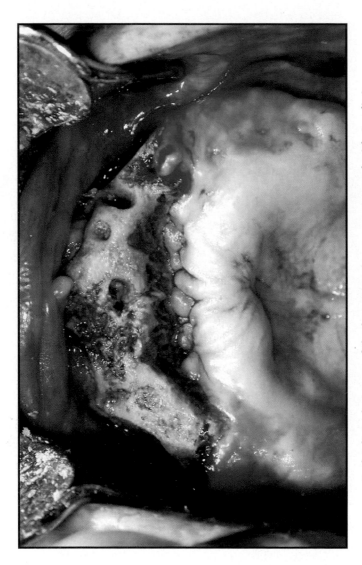

Early clinical picture of the lower jaw in woman treated with Aredia® and Zometa® for 24 months (48 years old, breast cancer)

increased risk of oral infection—precisely what is seen in women taking bisphosphonates who develop ONJ.

More than 2,000 cases of bisphosphonate-induced ONJ have been reported since 2003. In August 2009, a class action suit was brought against Merck, the pharmaceutical company responsible for Fosamax®, the most widely prescribed of the bisphosphonates. Merck has been accused of failing to adequately warn that this patent medicine may cause ONJ—a highly significant failure for those who have developed ONJ after taking Fosamax® since the condition is extremely difficult to live with, persistent, and responds poorly, if at all, to conventional treatments.

No one, not even Merck, is disputing the growing numbers of reports of ONJ in individuals taking Fosamax® and other bisphosphonates. Merck has received well over 1,000 reports from people who developed the condition after Fosamax® use. Merck claims, however, that the relationship between ONJ and Fosamax® is not a causal one, despite the fact that internal Merck documents and email comments made by one of Merck's own scientists, Dr. Donald B. Kimmel, indicate that bisphosphonates cause ONJ.

In 2005, Dr. Kimmel, who was their director of molecular endocrinology, warned that the severe reduction in bone remodeling caused by the bisphosphonate patent medicines is likely to reduce the jaw's natural ability to heal, and that placing too much of a healing demand on patients treated with bisphosphonates can lead to the death of the jaw bone.[11] Merck claims this was just one of "various theories" Kimmel examined when investigating how ONJ might develop.

One data point is uncontestable—ONJ incidence is increasing and occurs most frequently in older women taking bisphosphonates who have undergone dental work.[12] Merck estimates ONJ occurs in 1.6 individuals per 100,000 taking oral bisphosphonates, but a Kaiser Permanente survey found ONJ occurred in roughly 1 in 1,000 respondents who were still or had previously taken these patent medicines.[13] And new reports of ONJ are appearing in the medical journals virtually every month. As of May 10, 2010, more than 1,100 articles discussing bone death related to bisphosphonate use had been published in the peer-reviewed medical literature. These footnotes, in addition to the others in this section, provide just a tiny selection of some of the recent reports.[14] When we started tracking this, we would see one or two reports every few months. Now, we see several every week!

How Bisphosphonates Cause ONJ

Bisphosphonates accumulate in bones, particularly in the jawbone, and inhibit the bone's natural ability to repair everyday damage by about 90%.[15] The very unpleasant consequences are first apparent in the jaw rather than other bones for several reasons.[16] Bisphosphonates concentrate in the jaw bones because these bones have a greater blood supply than other bones and a faster bone turnover rate, due both to the daily trauma resulting from chewing and the presence of teeth, both of which make daily bone remodeling necessary around the *periodontal ligament*, the ligament that attaches the tooth to its socket in the jawbone.

Many Dentists Will Not Treat Women Taking Bisphosphonates

Even short-term use of oral bisphosphonates significantly increases risk of ONJ following dental work, particularly surgical dental procedures such as root canals or extractions. Sixty percent of all reported cases of ONJ have occurred after dental surgery to treat infections, with the remaining 40% related to infection, denture trauma, or other physical trauma.

In medical circles, Cochrane Reviews are known to be the best single source of scientific evidence about the effects of healthcare interventions. In a Cochrane Review, researchers evaluate the combined results of virtually all the best studies on a topic using rigorous methods carefully designed to prevent bias and errors in interpretation. A Cochrane review of bisphosphonate-related ONJ found that an age of 60 years or older, female sex, and previous invasive dental treatment were the common characteristics of patients taking bisphosphonates who developed ONJ.[17]

Since the primary target population for bisphosphonate use is postmenopausal women, many of whom are 60 or older and, as they age, are increasingly likely to need some kind of invasive dental procedure, these risk traits for ONJ with bisphosphonate use are far too common for comfort. In fact, they are so common that the American Dental Association has warned dentists to avoid "invasive dental procedures" in patients on IV bisphosphonates and to take a "conservative" approach to dental procedures for patients taking oral bisphosphonates.

The American Dental Association's updated recommendations for managing patients on oral bisphosphonates, released December 2008,[18] added a recommendation to dentists to protect *themselves* by consulting with an attorney to develop an informed consent form for patients taking bisphosphonates that will be certain to satisfy the criteria of the state in which they practice. Many dentists are becoming increasingly reluctant to perform any type of dental work on women taking these patent medicines.[19]

No Cure Exists for ONJ

A key reason for dentists' concern is that bisphosphonate-related ONJ is extremely difficult to treat. Affected individuals usually have no symptoms until dying bone becomes infected. Initial symptoms include numbness, heaviness, swelling, pain and infection in the jaw, and loosening of the teeth. Open sores or lesions develop that frequently do not respond to conventional treatments, including debridement (the removal of dead or infected tissue), antibiotics, and hyperbaric oxygen therapy.

Increasing patients' risk of ONJ by prescribing bisphosphonates is far from trivial since, currently, *no definitive cure exists*.[20] Most treatment is only palliative, providing some pain relief without restoring health, and the condition is associated with significant impaired eating ability, pain and disfigurement, resulting in greatly compromised quality of life.[21]

Bisphosphonates Promote Chronic Oral Infections

Bisphosphonates also contribute to chronic oral infections. Research published in the *Journal of Oral Maxillofacial Surgery* found a direct correlation between bisphosphonate use and the development of *microbial biofilms*, supersized bacterial colonies that cause chronic infections in affected bone.[22]

Bisphosphonates Increase Risk for Atrial Fibrillation

A number of recent studies, including a meta-analysis of four studies involving more than 26,000 postmenopausal women, have now reported that bisphosphonates increase risk for "serious atrial fibrillation"—that is, an erratic, irregular heartbeat, by more than 150%.[23] Over the last 20 years, atrial fibrillation has become the most commonly encountered cardiac arrhythmia in clinical practice, accounting for the majority of arrhythmia-related hospital admissions and greatly increasing risk of stroke.[24]

A study published in the *New England Journal of Medicine* in 2007 found Fosamax® increased likelihood of serious atrial fibrillation events by 150%.[25] Data from a more recent study, published in the journal *Menopause* in 2009, show that Fosamax® caused a more than twofold (or 200%) increase in risk for atrial fibrillation.[26] Yet another study, published in the *Archives of Internal Medicine* in 2008, estimates that 3% of *all* atrial fibrillation cases that have occurred since the bisphosphonate patent medicines received FDA approval over 16 years ago may have been due to bisphosphonate (specifically, Fosamax® [alendronate]) therapy, and warns that bisphosphonate use should be closely monitored in populations at high risk of serious adverse effects from atrial fibrillation, which includes patients with heart failure, coronary artery disease, or diabetes.[27]

In other words, those at risk for serious side effects from bisphosphonates include not only women aged 60 and older who might need dental work, but also anyone with heart disease or diabetes—or more than one-third of the entire US adult population.

Bisphosphonates: A Long List of Other Adverse Side Effects

Numerous other adverse effects have also been reported, including:[28]

- **Erosions and ulcerations of the esophagus (throat) and severe damage to the lining of the gastrointestinal tract**

  These are the key reasons for the detailed procedure necessary for taking these patent medicines, which must be consumed with a full 6-8 oz. glass of ordinary (not mineral) water, first thing in the morning after getting out of bed, and at least 30 minutes before ingesting any other food, beverage, or medication, during which time the patient must consume an additional 2 oz. of water and cannot lie down until at least 30 minutes later after food has been consumed.

  The results of the 1-year findings in the Prospective Observational Scientific Study

Investigating Bone Loss Experience in the US (POSSIBLE US), published April 2010, showed that 20% of women taking bisphosphonates reported gastrointestinal side effects when they began participating in the study. Side effects frequently became so severe that when the women were questioned again after 6 months, those using bisphosphonates were 139% more likely to have stopped taking the patent medicines.[29]

■ Esophageal Cancer

People who take oral bisphosphonates for bone disease for more than five years may be doubling their risk of developing esophageal cancer, according to a study published September 2010 in the *British Medical Journal*.[30] The researchers analyzed data from the UK General Practice Research Database, which includes patient records for around six million people. They focused on men and women aged over 40 years, identifying 2,954 cases of esophageal cancer. Each case was compared with five controls matched for age, sex, general practice, and observation period. People with 10 prescriptions for bisphosphonates—or who had been prescribed bisphosphonates over a period of five years—had nearly double the risk of esophageal cancer compared with people with no bisphosphonate prescriptions.

- **Influenza-like illness**

  Bisphosphonates may cause a flu-like syndrome, particularly in the early phase of treatment. Onset is sudden, and symptoms commonly include fever, shivering, chills, dry cough, loss of appetite, body aches, and nausea.[31]

- **Myalgia (severe muscle pain)**

  In clinical trials, approximately 4% of patients treated with Fosamax® (alendronate) developed muscle, bone, or joint pain. The time to onset of severe muscle pain varied from one day to several months after starting treatment. When patients stopped taking alendronate, their myalgia usually—but not always—went away.[32]

- **Deterioration of kidney function and kidney failure**

  Studies have shown the bisphosphonates, especially zoledronic acid (sold under the trade names of Zometa® and Reclast®), are toxic to the kidneys. The peer-reviewed medical studies show kidney function is harmed in 8.8–15.2% of patients given zoledronic acid.[33]

- **Symptomatic hypocalcemia (too little calcium in the circulation)**

  This can cause seizures, gastric achlorhydria (too little stomach acid to be able to properly digest food), dementia, dangerously low blood pressure, bronchospasm (when the bands of muscle around the airways tighten uncontrollably, as in asthma), and heart failure.

  Reports of symptomatic hypocalcemia are increasing in patients receiving the latest additions to the bisphosphonates, Reclast® and Aclasta®. These patent medicines, which contain zoledronic acid and must be given intravenously, are being promoted as a more "convenient" way to prevent osteoporosis since they are so potent, so poisonous to the normal functioning of osteoclasts, that they are administered only once a year.[34]

■ **Bone stress fracture**

Wait a minute, isn't this what these patent medicines are supposed to prevent? The peer-reviewed research, published in top medical journals on this adverse side effect of bisphosphonates, is discussed next, and proves that bisphosphonates actually *increase* fracture risk.[35]

Bisphosphonates *Increase* Fracture Risk

Starting in 2005, studies began appearing showing that bisphosphonates' suppression of normal bone remodeling increases fracture risk in as little as 2½ years.

In 2005, in what is called a "case series" in the medical journals, physicians working at the same hospital reported on nine patients who, after 3 to 8 years on Fosamax®, experienced fractures "while performing normal daily activities such as walking, standing, or turning around." In six of these patients, all of whom were told to continue to take Fosamax® after their fracture, healing was delayed, taking from 3 months to *2 years longer* than the time normally expected for healing.[36]

A case report in 2007 alerted physicians that two hospitals had seen 13 women (average age 66.9 years) who suffered thighbone fractures with minimal or no trauma—in other words, during normal daily activities—during a 10-month period (May 2005 to February 2006). Nine of these women had been taking Fosamax®, several for as little as 2½ years.[37]

In another case series, published in 2008, researchers looked at the records of patients admitted to a Level 1 trauma center over a five-year period. They found that low-energy thighbone fractures (i.e., fractures occurring during normal daily activities) with a specific, uncommon *transverse* (crosswise) pattern were associated with Fosamax® use. This is especially concerning since the thighbone is the thickest, strongest bone in the body.

Seventy patients with this type of low-energy thighbone fracture (59 women, 11 men, average age 74.7 years) were identified. Of these, 25 were taking Fosamax®, and 19 of them suffered a low-energy thighbone fracture with the same unusual pattern. In contrast, only one patient not being treated with Fosamax® had this fracture pattern, which translates to a 98% increased risk for this uncommon type of fracture in patients taking Fosamax®.

While most of the patients experiencing this uncommon type of thigh bone fracture had been taking Fosamax® longer than those who did not have this type of fracture (6.9 years versus 2.5 years, respectively), one patient in this study had been taking Fosamax® for less than 4 years. Thus, although it is clearly true that the longer a woman takes a bisphosphonate, the greater her accumulation of brittle bone and risk of fracture during normal daily activity, in some people, unhealthy bone accumulates much more quickly.

Researchers think that the increased risk of thighbone fracture during normal activity seen with Fosamax® is a result of the accumulation of tiny stress fractures whose healing is prevented by the patent medicine's suppression of osteoclast activity and microdamage repair.[38] In lab animals, Fosamax® increased the number of microcracks by 2- to 7-fold, and a study involving 66 postmenopausal women with osteoporosis found 30% more microdamage in the bones of those taking Fosamax®.[39]

In 2009, physicians at the University Hospitals of Geneva, Switzerland, voiced concerns to the Swiss National Pharmacovigilance Centre about bisphosphonates' long-term harmful effects after admitting a series of eight patients who had been treated with bisphosphonates to their regional hospital for low-energy thighbone fractures. Some of these patients had been on Fosamax® for as little as 16 months; one had been on Boniva® only 4 months.[40]

Numerous papers are now reporting that bisphosphonates' repression of bone turnover actually promotes the accumulation of microcracks and the occurrence of unexpected stress fractures, characteristically at the subtrochanter of the femur (below the trochanter but in the upper part of the body of the thigh bone, see images on following pages).[41] In some especially unfortunate individuals, these fragility fractures are occurring in both femurs simultaneously!*[42]

The question researchers are now asking is, "How long can a person take bisphosphonates before these patent medicines *cause* a fragility fracture?" The current estimate is a maximum of five years.[43]

In 2008, the FDA questioned Merck about increasing reports of femur fractures spontaneously occurring in women taking Fosamax® during normal daily activities. It took Merck more than a year to respond, but 16 months later, they very quietly added "low energy femoral shaft and sub-trochanteric fractures" to the list of possible side effects in the patent medicine's package insert.

According to ABC News senior health and medical editor, Dr. Richard Besser, neither

---

* The many endnotes listed in this citation are just a representative sampling, taken from among dozens of papers now appearing in the peer-reviewed medical literature on this highly negative outcome of bisphosphonate use.

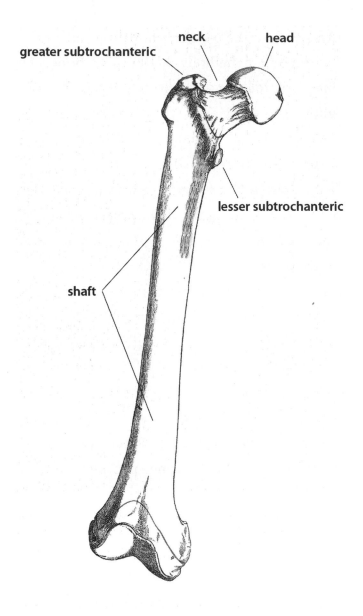

Diagram of femur.

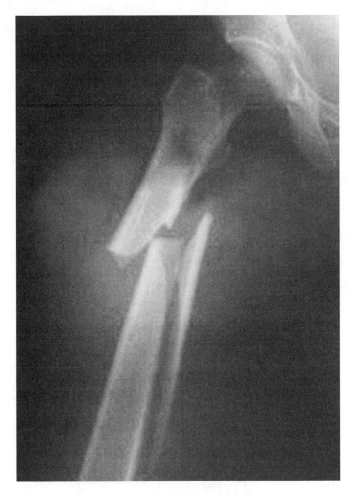

X-ray* showing fracture in the upper half of Dr. Jennifer Schneider's right femur caused by a subway car jolt following 7 years of Fosamax® treatment.

---

* Courtesy of Dr. Schneider, from *Stay Young and Sexy with Bio-Identical Hormone Replacement* (Petaluma, CA: Smart Publications, 2010).

Merck nor the FDA made any effort to inform doctors or the public that all the bisophospho-nates—including not just Fosamax®, but Acto-nel®, Boniva®, and Reclast®—*cause* fractures. Both the FDA and Merck refused a request by ABC News for an interview, although the FDA announced in a drug safety communication issued March 10, 2010, that they would look into whether there is an increased risk of "atyp-ical subtrochanteric femur fractures" in women using bisphosphonates.[44]

Following their review of all available data on bisphosphonate use, on October 13, 2010, FDA issued a bulletin[45] warning patients and health care providers that all the bisphosphonates pre-scribed for osteoporosis increase risk for atypi-cal thigh bone fractures and announced that the bisphosphonates must change their labeling and include a Medication Guide to ensure physi-cian and patient awareness of this risk. The FDA bulletin includes two recommendations: (1) that health care professionals reevaluate the need for continued bisphosphonate use in patients who have been taking these patent medicines for longer than five years, and (2) that patients taking bisphosphonates report any new thigh or groin pain to their health care provider and be evaluated for a possible femur fracture. Patients and health care professionals are asked to report side effects with bisphosphonate use to the FDA's MedWatch Adverse Event Reporting program at www.fda.gov/MedWatch or by calling (800) 332-1088.

Not only do the bisphosphonates increase risk of femur fracture, but they also greatly increase the likelihood that the broken bone will not heal. In June 2009, a study involving 19,731 patients with thighbone fractures was conducted at Harvard Medical School to evaluate the effects of bisphosphonates on bones' ability to heal. Bisphosphonate use more than doubled the risk of "nonunion"—medical jargon meaning the bone had become incapable of re-joining and could not heal.[46]

What we are now seeing is simply the result of the fact that many women have now been taking bisphosphonates long enough to do very serious damage to their bones. Class action lawsuits brought as a result of bisphosphonate-related osteonecrosis of the jaw are now underway on three continents and are thought to be "a worrying precursor for millions of other consumers who will soon reach the five-year oral half-life of bisphosphonates," which is when the adverse effects of these patent medicines typically begin to become apparent.[47]

Reports of spontaneous fractures will continue to increase until many more class action lawsuits have been brought against the patent medicine companies responsible. Don't wait until the FDA and Merck are forced to acknowledge the harm done to millions of women. If you are taking a bisphosphonate, stop! If your doctor is telling you to start taking any of these patent medicines, refuse—and give him or her a copy of this book, so you can get on a safe bone-building program that works!

Bisphosphonates and Breast Cancer

In women with advanced breast cancer that has metastasized to bone, some research suggests that bisphosphonates may be of sufficient benefit to offset their risks *if used short term.*

Cancer cells produce osteoclast-activating factors that play a role in the pathogenesis of bone cancer. Since bisphosphonates poison osteoclasts, these patent medicines may be helpful *in women with advanced breast cancer that has metastasized to bone.*

In some studies, the IV bisphosphonate zoledronate (marketed under the trade names Aclasta®, Reclast®, Zometa®, Zomera®), has been shown to reduce bone pain, help prevent fracture and spinal cord compression, and improve quality of life. However, with the increasing use of bisphosphonates for metastatic bone disease has also come to light the fact that these patent medicines have toxic effects, including ONJ,*

---

* See previous images on pages 17 and 18.

that greatly promote morbidity in patients with advanced cancer.[48]

Since even in women without cancer, bisphosphonate therapy, especially with zoledronte (marketed under the trade names Aclasta®, Reclast®, Zometa®, Zomera®) taken for longer than two years, greatly increases risk of ONJ, medical authorities do not recommend the use of bisphosphonates for women with early stage breast cancer.

Oral bisphosphonates have been used to help lessen bone loss in postmenopausal women with estrogen-receptor positive breast cancer who have been prescribed patent medicines called aromatase-inhibitors. *Aromatase* is an enzyme involved in the formation of the most potent form of estrogen, *estradiol*, which can contribute to the progression of hormone positive breast cancer. However, since estrogen plays an important role in preventing excessive bone loss, aromatase-inhibiting patent medicines also promote bone loss, greatly increasing risk of osteoporosis.

Recently, two studies have suggested that bisphosphonates may be linked to a reduction in breast cancer risk. One study using data from the Women's Health Initiative found 32% fewer cases of invasive breast cancer in women who used bisphosphonates. The second, an Israeli study, found that more than five years of bisphosphonate use was associated with a 29% reduction in risk of postmenopausal breast cancer. Whether these associations are simply coincidence or really indicate that bisphosphonates may help reduce breast cancer risk remains unknown. All the experts agree that more studies are necessary to find out.[49]

But why should women even consider risking the serious side effects clearly associated with all the bisphosphonates when there are completely safe and effective ways to reduce breast cancer risk—and improve overall health—using research-proven diet, supplement, and lifestyle choices with *no* toxic side effects?

Even in women with breast cancer, supplementation with the naturally occurring mineral, strontium, which not only reduces bone resorption but stimulates the formation of healthy new bone (especially when combined with calcium and other nutrients necessary for bone re-mineralization, such as vitamins D and K_2), does a much better job of building healthy bone than bisphosphonates any day! [50]

Say Bye-Bye to Bisphosphonates!

Since bone is constantly remodeling throughout our lives, any therapy used to promote bone health in aging women must be one a woman can rely upon for the rest of her life. Obviously, it makes little sense to take a patent medicine that, at best, only conserves old, worn-out bone, and may increase fracture risk within as little as four months!

Even a quick look at the many serious risks associated with taking bisphosphonates, especially when combined with the fact that these patent medicines actually increase your likelihood of developing bones so brittle they break during normal daily activities, provides sufficient reason to question the advisability of relying on these patent medicines to prevent osteoporosis!

A substantial amount of top quality, peer-reviewed research shows that the balance between osteoclasts' demolition of old, worn-out bone and osteoblasts' reconstruction of healthy, new bone can be restored safely without recourse to dangerous and expensive patent medicines.

What we need to do is identify and control the factors that are causing our osteoclasts to become hyperactive, so they remove too much bone, and to be sure we are providing our osteoblasts with an adequate supply of all the materials they need to build new bone. Once this is accomplished, our bodies will happily set about doing what they are born already programmed to do—provide us with strong bones for life, naturally.

PART 3

What Increases Your Risk for Osteoporosis?

CHAPTER 3

What You Don't Know Can Give You Osteoporosis

IN THE FOLLOWING CHAPTERS, WE LOOK AT THE KEY factors affecting bone remodeling and the nutrients our bodies need to build healthy bones. You'll find it easy to identify which of these factors applies to you, and which nutrients your bones need that your current diet and supplement program is not adequately supplying.

Once you have recognized what *you*—not some imaginary "average" person—need, you can take the steps necessary to protect and enhance the health of your bones. Safeguard and nourish your bones, and they will repay you by beautifully supporting you throughout a long and vibrant life.

Are You Sure You're Getting Enough Calcium?

As we get older, we normally lose a tiny amount of bone each year. Not getting enough daily calcium can greatly accelerate our rate of bone loss.

Although most of us think we get plenty of calcium, surprisingly, a review of data from the most recent NHANES (National Health and Nutrition Examination Survey) found that 60% of Americans are not getting enough calcium, even when including both food and supplements, to meet current recommendations for adequate calcium intake.[51]

Recommendations for adequate intake (AI) of calcium were issued by the Institute of Medicine at the National Academy of Sciences in 1998. For those most at risk for osteoporosis—women approaching or currently experiencing their transition through menopause—these recommendations are:

- 31–50 years: 1,000 mg
- 51+ years: 1,200 mg
- Postmenopausal women not taking hormone replacement therapy: 1,500 mg

To determine whether you are, in fact, consuming enough calcium to maintain your bones' health, you'll want to take a look at your typical diet and, if you are taking supplements, the amount of calcium they contain.

On the next page is a list of foods rich in calcium, and the amount of calcium a typical serving of each provides. You can easily check whether you are getting enough calcium. For 5 to 7 days, keep a food and supplement diary each day, then look to see how much calcium you're really getting.

I Need More than Calcium to Prevent Osteoporosis?

Yes, most definitely! Normal bone metabolism is an intricate interplay among more than two dozen nutrients, including, in addition to calcium, the vitamins D, K, B_6, B_{12}, and folate, and

FOODS RICH IN CALCIUM

Food	Serving Size	Calcium
Cow's milk,* 2% fat	1 cup	297 mg
Yogurt, low-fat	1 cup	447 mg
Cottage cheese, 1% fat	1 cup	100 mg
Mozarella cheese, part-skim	1 ounce	183 mg
Swiss cheese	1 ounce	265 mg
Goat milk	1 cup	326 mg
Salmon, canned	4 ounces	300 mg
Sardines, canned with bones	2 ounces	240 mg
Spinach, steamed	1 cup	245 mg
Collard greens, steamed	1 cup	226 mg
Kale, steamed	1 cup	94 mg
Romaine lettuce	2 cups	40 mg
Broccoli, steamed	1 cup	75 mg
Green beans	1 cup	57 mg
Cabbage, shredded, steamed	1 cup	46 mg
Sesame seeds	1/4 cup	351 mg
Tofu	4 ounces	100 mg
Orange	1 raw	52 mg
Almonds	1 ounce (about 20 nuts)	70 mg

* However, don't rely on cow's milk as your primary source of calcium. The nearly 78,000 woman *Harvard Nurses Study* determined that osteoporosis risk actually increased with increased use of milk and dairy products.

the minerals boron, magnesium, and phosphorous. What you need to know about each one of
these nutrients to build and maintain healthy
bone is laid out in the section "Strong Bones for
Life, Naturally."* Our agenda here is to convince
you that your bones need a good deal more than
calcium to stay strong.

As mentioned earlier, our hormones play
key roles in maintaining healthy bone. In
women, estrogen regulates osteoclasts, keeping them under control, so they only remove
dead demineralized bone, and progesterone
helps activate osteoblasts, which build new
bone. Levels of both hormones begin to decline
several years before menopause, during the
time in a woman's life called *perimenopause*
("peri" = around).

While the average age at which perimenopause begins is 47.5 years in the Western world,
for some women this transition to menopause
begins in their early 40s. Average length of time
during perimenopause is about four years, with

---

* See page 133.

menopause most often occurring around the age of 51 (or 49 in women who smoke).[52]

In men, hormones also play a key role in maintaining bone mass. Testosterone's importance in maintaining bone mass in men is not as well understood as the roles played by estrogen and progesterone in women, but the androgens (male hormones) are known to be involved in the development of osteoblasts, and some testosterone is metabolized into estradiol, the most potent form of estrogen, which also plays an important role in men's healthy bone remodeling.[53]

As men age, their testosterone levels decline, although not as early or as abruptly as women's levels of estrogen and progesterone do. However, by age 60, virtually all men have experienced a drop in their levels of male hormones or androgens, which increases the rate at which men lose bone. Androgen deprivation therapy, which is commonly used in the treatment of prostate cancer, results in a 3% to 5% yearly loss in bone mineral density and is well known to promote osteoporosis in men.[54]

In addition to the nutrients noted above and our sex hormones, a variety of genetic and lifestyle factors affect our body's ability to maintain a healthy balance between bone resorption and formation. Let's take a look at the most important of these next.

I Need Stomach Acid to Absorb Calcium?

Yes! Despite the fact that TV commercials tell us that heartburn and indigestion are caused by too much stomach acid, *too little* stomach acid not only results in the same symptoms (heartburn or reflux from half-digested food backing up the throat, bloating, belching, and gas), but promotes osteoporosis because, without sufficient stomach acid, we cannot absorb calcium.

In order for calcium to be absorbed in the intestines, it must first be made soluble (able to be dissolved) and ionized (made to have fewer electrons) by stomach acid. Studies have found that almost 40% of postmenopausal women are severely deficient in stomach acid![55]

Not surprisingly, decreased stomach acid is common in both women and men who frequently take antacids to relieve heartburn or indigestion. Over-the-counter antacids, such as Maalox®, Tums®, or Rolaids®, neutralize acid already present in the stomach, while the acid-blocking patent medicines, including the H2 blockers (e.g., Pepcid®, Tagament®, Axid®) and the proton pump inhibitors (e.g., Prilosec®, Nexium®, Prevacid®), suppress the stomach's ability to produce acid. Among the acid-blocking patent medicines, H2 blockers are less harmful to bone than the proton pump inhibitors because H2 blockers only decrease the amount of stomach acid produced, while proton pump inhibitors completely shut down the stomach's ability to produce stomach acid.

Relying on these patent medicines instead of taking a look at the diet and lifestyle habits that are the *cause* of our upset stomachs is like turning off the fire alarm and going back to bed while the house continues to burn down. Not only do all the antacid patent medicines fail to address the reasons for our indigestion problems, but they promote other ones, including osteoporosis.

When we turn to supplements to ensure we are getting enough calcium, having enough stomach acid can be especially important. Calcium carbonate, the least expensive and therefore the most commonly used form of calcium in nutritional supplements, is neither soluble nor ionized. Individuals who produce little stomach acid only absorb about 4% of an oral dose of calcium carbonate, and even persons who produce normal amounts of stomach acid absorb only 22% of an oral dose of this form of supplemental calcium.[56]

Fortunately, even patients with low stomach acid will absorb much more—about 45%—of the calcium from supplements providing calcium in the form of *calcium citrate*.[57] In a number of studies involving healthy women, women with low stomach acid production, and women who had undergone gastric bypass surgery (gastric bypass restricts food intake, thus lowering the amount of *all* vitamins and minerals, including calcium, available to be absorbed from the digestive tract), calcium citrate has been shown to be a much more effective means of delivering calcium into the bloodstream than calcium carbonate.[58]

Regardless of whether you suspect your production of stomach acid is low or you have no problems digesting your food (and therefore are producing enough stomach acid to do so), if you are taking a supplement containing calcium carbonate, be sure to take it with a meal to maximize your production of stomach acid and your ability to absorb its calcium.[59] If you're uncertain, why not just switch from calcium carbonate to calcium citrate?

Is Your Diet Leaching Calcium from Your Bones?

A slightly alkaline body chemistry, which is what is seen in individuals whose diet includes lots of plant foods (vegetables, fruits, beans, whole grains, nuts and seeds, etc.), is required for good bone health. A diet high in animal protein results in an acidic body chemistry, which our bodies attempt to buffer by withdrawing alkaline minerals, i.e., calcium, from our bones.

Research has very clearly shown that a diet too high in protein greatly increases the amount of calcium released from our bones and excreted in the urine. In a study that looked at the effects of diets containing varying amounts of protein on the bones of women with osteoporosis, raising their daily protein intake from 47 to 142 grams *doubled* the amount of calcium lost in their urine.[60] This is one reason why vegetarian diets (both those that include dairy products and eggs as well as vegan diets) are associated with a lower risk of developing osteoporosis.[61]

How Much Protein Do YOU Need?

Three steps are necessary to figure this out, each of which is explained below. Here is what you will be doing: first, you'll determine your ideal weight. Then you'll convert your ideal weight from pounds to kilograms. And lastly, you'll multiply your ideal weight in kilograms by 0.8 to determine the number of grams of protein *your* body needs each day. If you do not want to bother with this, the chart below will give you a reasonable estimate of how many grams of protein you need each day.

Step One: Determining Your Ideal Weight

Your daily protein requirements are based on your *ideal* weight, not your current weight. Ideal weight for a woman 5 feet (60 inches) tall is 100 pounds. If you are taller than 5 feet, add 5 pounds for each additional inch in your height over 60 inches. So, for example, if you are 5 feet 6 inches tall, your ideal weight would be 5 feet (100 pounds) plus 6 inches (5 pounds x 6 inches = 30 pounds) for a total of 130 pounds.

DAILY PROTEIN REQUIREMENTS BY WEIGHT

Height	Ideal Wt. in Lbs.	Ideal Wt. in Kgs.	Grams of Protein Needed
5'2"	110.00	49.5	39.6
5'3"	115.00	51.75	41.4
5'4"	120.00	54	43.2
5'5"	125.00	56.25	45
5'6"	130.00	58.5	46.8
5'7"	135.00	60.75	48.6
5'8"	140.00	63	50.4
5'9"	145.00	65.25	52.2

Step Two: Convert Your Ideal Weight in Pounds to Kilograms

One pound = 0.45 kilograms, so to convert your weight in pounds to kilograms multiply your weight in pounds by 0.45. For example, 130 pounds multiplied by 0.45 = 58.5 kilograms.

Step Three: Multiply Your Weight in Kilograms by 0.8

The US Recommended Daily Allowance (RDA) for protein intake is 0.8 grams of protein per kilogram of ideal body weight each day. To find the number of grams of protein you need daily, multiply your weight in kilograms by 0.8. Thus, for the 5 foot 6 inch woman in our example, whose ideal weight is 130 pounds or 58.5 kilograms, the calculation is 58.5 x 0.8 = 46.8 grams. Unfortunately, diets containing significantly more protein than is needed are quite common in the United States. Analysis of NHANES (National Health and Nutrition Examination Survey) data show that daily protein intakes ranging from 91 to 113 grams are typical in the majority of adults (19 and older), and decrease to amounts that still remain quite a bit higher than needed—around 66 to 83 grams per day—in many elders 71 years or older.[62]

On the other hand, somewhere between 15 to 38% of adult men and 27 to 41% of adult women have dietary protein intakes *below* the RDA.[63] A diet too low in protein has been associated with reduced absorption of calcium from the intestines, which researchers are concerned may also increase bone loss.[64]

To determine *your* typical protein intake, keep a food diary for three to five days (if you kept a food diary to check that you were getting enough calcium, you can use that here as well), then use the list of protein-rich foods listed in the following table to check and see if you are supplying your body with sufficient protein to meet your needs—but not overdoing it.

FOODS RICH IN PROTEIN

Food	Serving Size	Protein
Cod, baked/broiled	4 ounces	26 grams
Tuna, yellowfin, baked/broiled	4 ounces	34 grams
Snapper, baked/broiled	4 ounces	30 grams
Halibut, baked/broiled	4 ounces	30 grams
Scallops, baked/broiled	4 ounces	23 grams
Shrimp, steamed/boiled	4 ounces	24 grams
Sardines, canned	1 can, 3.75 ounces	23 grams
Salmon, baked/broiled	4 ounces	29 grams
Chicken breast, roasted	4 ounces	33 grams
Turkey breast, roasted	4 ounces	33 grams
Beef tenderloin, lean, broiled	4 ounces	32 grams
Lamb loin, roasted	4 ounces	30 grams
Calf's liver, braised	4 ounces	25 grams
Egg, whole, boiled	1	6 grams
Tofu	4 ounces	10 grams
Tempeh, cooked	4 ounces	21 grams
Soybeans, cooked	1 cup	29 grams
Split peas, cooked	1 cup	16 grams
Kidney beans, cooked	1 cup	15 grams
Lima beans, cooked	1 cup	15 grams
Black beans, cooked	1 cup	15 grams
Navy beans, cooked	1 cup	15 grams
Pinto beans, cooked	1 cup	14 grams
Garbanzo beans, cooked	1 cup	15 grams
Lentils, cooked	1 cup	18 grams

Food	Serving Size	Protein
Peanuts	1/4 cup	10 grams
Pumpkin seeds	1/4 cup	9 grams
Cow's milk	1 cup	8 grams
Yogurt, low-fat	1 cup	13 grams
Cottage cheese	3 ounces	14 grams
Mozzarella cheese, part skim	1 ounce	7 grams
Cheddar	1 ounce	8 grams
Cheddar, low fat	1 ounce	10 grams
Feta	1 ounce	5 grams
Parmesan	1 ounce	8 grams
Oats, whole grain, cooked	1 cup	6 grams
Bread, whole wheat	1 slice	3 grams
Bread, white	1 slice	2.5 grams
Pasta, whole wheat, boiled	3 ounces	9 grams
Pasta, refined flour, boiled	3 ounces	7 grams
Rice, brown	7 ounces	5 grams
Rice, white	7 ounces	5 grams
Asparagus	3.5 ounces	3 grams
Broccoli	3.5 ounces	3 grams
Cauliflower	3.5 ounces	3 grams
Spinach	3.5 ounces	2 grams
Tomato	3.5 ounces	2 grams
Yam	3.5 ounces	2 grams
Beet	3.5 ounces	2 grams
Onion	3.5 ounces	2 grams
Sweet corn	3.5 ounces	2.5 grams
Mushrooms	3.5 ounces	2 grams

Refined Sugars Make Your Belly Fat but Your Bones Skinny

Consumption of refined sugars, such as the high fructose corn syrup now added to virtually every processed packaged food and beverage, promotes acidic body chemistry. Similar to what happens when you eat too much animal protein, when your diet is loaded with refined sugars, your urinary excretion of calcium increases.

The average American consumes 125 grams of sucrose (table sugar) and 50 grams of corn syrup each day in processed foods, which also contain other refined simple sugars (e.g., dextrose). (Since neither of your authors consumes any sucrose or corn syrup at all, there are at least one or two people who must be consuming 250 grams [almost 9 ounces] of sucrose and 100 grams [approximately 3½ ounces] of corn syrup daily, for a grand total of over three-quarters of a pound of just these two simple sugars daily!) And that doesn't even count carbonated beverages (sodas) high in both refined sugars and phosphates, both of which promote bone loss.[65] Our genes, which have changed only about 0.01% since the Paleolithic era when the only refined sugar humans encountered was a very occasional bit of honey, are not equipped to handle this sugar tsunami.

While 99.9% of our genetic profile is still Paleolithic, 70% of the average caloric intake of Americans comes from food products that did not even exist for our Paleolithic ancestors, for example, cookies, French fries, corn chips, or soft drinks. Somehow, our ancestors not only survived but evolved. Humans today may not be faring as well. Research published in the *New England Journal of Medicine* indicates that the current generation of children in the US is likely to live shorter lives than their parents, largely because the rapid rise in obesity, if unchecked, will shorten life spans by as much as five years.[66]

Soft Drinks Are Hard on Bones

Soft drinks hit your bones with a double whammy since they dose you not only with refined sugars, but large amounts of phosphates, and no calcium. When phosphate levels are high, and calcium levels are low, calcium is—you guessed it—once again pulled out of your bones to restore balance. The "average" American consumes 15 ounces of soda pop every day.[67] Even if you drink "diet soda," your bones are still being assaulted by phosphates.

Greens Give the Go-Ahead for Great Bones; Their Absence Slams the Brakes on Bone-Building

Green leafy vegetables are packed with all the vitamins and minerals necessary for bone health, including calcium, vitamin K, boron, and magnesium. Unfortunately, very few Americans are eating leafy greens.

According to research conducted by the Center for Disease Control and Prevention, adults in the US average, at best, no more than 3.4 servings per day of fruits and vegetables *combined*.[68] Data collected by the second National Health and Nutrition Examination Survey showed that only 27% of Americans were eating at least three servings of vegetables daily (and this included potatoes, of which the vast majority were consumed in the form of French fries or potato chips).[69]

Since a serving of vegetables is just one-half cup (the equivalent of five broccoli florets, ten baby carrots, or half a baked sweet potato) or one cup of leafy greens (such as lettuce, spinach, kale, collards, or Swiss chard), these statistics go a long way towards explaining why osteoporosis is so common. Our bodies simply cannot build bone unless we provide them with the necessary ingredients to do so. It's like asking someone to whip up an omelet with no eggs.

"Bs" for Better Bones

The B vitamins—vitamin B_6, vitamin B_{12}, folate, and riboflavin—are involved in a cellular process called *methylation*, which jump starts and stops many vital processes in the body. Methylation is so important to so many of the biochemical processes that support our life that it occurs throughout the body billions of times every second!

At one of the steps in the methylation cycle, the amino acid *methionine* must be converted into another amino acid called *cysteine*, and this conversion requires vitamin B_{12} and the activated forms of vitamin B_6 and folate. The activated forms of vitamin B_6 and folate are produced by an enzyme called *flavin adenine dinucleotide* or *FAD*, which requires riboflavin (vitamin B_2) as a necessary component (co-factor).

Why do you need to know about all of this? If any of these B vitamins are not available throughout the body in adequate amounts, the methylation cycle stops midway at the point where an intermediate product called *homocysteine* gets produced. And homocysteine is a very nasty, very inflammatory compound—the molecular equivalent of a terrorist with an acid-spray gun.

When levels of homocysteine get too high within our cells, it leaks into the bloodstream and wreaks all kinds of havoc throughout the body. In addition to promoting osteoporosis,[70] high levels of homocysteine are strongly linked to cardiovascular diseases including atherosclerosis, peripheral artery disease, heart attack, and stroke;[71]

neuropsychiatric diseases such as Alzheimer's dementia, Parkinson's disease, schizophrenia, and depression;[72] kidney disease;[73] rheumatoid arthritis;[74] and worsening the vascular complications associated with type 2 diabetes.[75]

Homocysteine harms bone, specifically, because concentrations of homocysteine—which, by the way, typically increase during and after menopause—interfere with collagen cross-linking, and this results in the production of a defective bone matrix.[76] In other words, the internal structure of bone built when homocysteine levels are high is defective.

The impact of high homocysteine levels on bone health can be quite significant. In one study involving 1,002 men and women whose average age was 75, those with high levels of homocysteine (>14 micromol/liter) had a 70% higher risk of hip fracture.[77]

B vitamin deficiencies are quite common in the US, and they typically increase with age. Even during childbearing years, women are at increased risk of B vitamin deficiency due to the widespread use of oral contraceptives, which lower blood levels of vitamins B_6 and B_{12}, putting premenopausal women at increased risk of cardiovascular disease.[78]

Among individuals 65 and older, the most recent NHANES data indicates that only 38% have adequate blood levels of folate.[79] A study involving one hundred and fifty-two consecutive outpatients, ages 65 to 99, found that 14.5% were deficient in B_{12}.[80] Large surveys in the US have repeatedly found that at least 6% of those aged 60 or older are vitamin B_{12} deficient and that the likelihood of deficiency increases with age, so that closer to 20% of Americans have marginal B_{12} levels in later life.[81] Incidence of deficiency is even higher in individuals with type 2 diabetes, due in part to the fact that metformin (a patent medicine that lowers blood sugar levels and is prescribed for people with type 2 diabetes) inhibits B_{12} absorption. A recent study of individuals with type 2 diabetes revealed that 22% were B_{12} deficient.[82]

Do You Have Enough of These Bs on Board?

Use the 5- to-7-day food diary you kept to esti-mate your calcium and protein intake to get an estimate of how much B_6, B_{12}, folate, and ribo-flavin your typical diet is giving you each day. If you are taking a multiple vitamin and mineral supplement, be sure to add in the B vitamins it supplies when you check to see if you are meet-ing your bones' needs for B vitamins.

Recommended daily intake of B vitamins for bone health:

- B_6: 50 milligrams
- B_{12}: 500 micrograms
- Folate: 2,000 micrograms
- Riboflavin: 50 milligrams

BEST FOOD SOURCES OF VITAMIN B_6 INCLUDE:

Food	Serving Size	Amount of B_6
Tuna, yellowfin, baked or broiled	4 ounces	1.18 mg
Cod, baked or broiled	4 ounces	0.52 mg
Snapper, baked or broiled	4 ounces	0.52 mg

Food	Serving Size	Amount of B6
Salmon, baked or broiled	4 ounces	0.52 mg
Halibut	4 ounces	0.45 mg
Chicken breast, roasted	4 ounces	0.64 mg
Turkey breast, roasted	4 ounces	0.54 mg
Spinach, raw	1 cup	0.44 mg
Banana	1	0.68 mg
Potato, baked with skin	1 cup	0.42 mg
Avocado slices	1 cup	0.41 mg
Green peas, boiled	1 cup	0.35 mg

BEST FOOD SOURCES OF VITAMIN B_{12} INCLUDE:

Food	Serving Size	Amount of B_{12}
Calves' liver, braised	4 ounces	41.39 mcg
Snapper, baked or broiled	4 ounces	3.97 mcg
Salmon, baked or broiled	4 ounces	3.25 mcg
Beef tenderloin, lean, broiled	4 ounces	2.92 mcg
Lamb loin, roasted	4 ounces	2.45 mcg
Halibut	4 ounces	1.55 mcg
Cod, baked or broiled	4 ounces	1.18 mcg
Yogurt, low-fat	1 cup	1.38 mcg
Cow's milk, 2%	1 cup	0.89 mcg
Egg, whole, boiled	1	0.49 mcg

BEST FOOD SOURCES OF RIBOFLAVIN INCLUDE:

Food	Serving Size	Amount of Riboflavin
Cow's milk, nonfat	8 ounces	0.6 mg
Cheese, Danish blue	1 ounce	0.6 mg
Cheese, Parmesan	1/3rd ounce	0.5 mg
Cheese, Cheddar	1 ounce	0.5 mg
Yogurt	6 ounces	0.2 mg
Beef sirloin	3 ounces	0.3 mg
Corn flakes, enriched	1 ounce	1.3 mg
Chicken liver	4 ounces	1.7 mg
Egg, boiled	1 large	0.5 mg
Almonds	10 nuts	0.9 mg
Cashews	10 nuts	0.2 mg
Walnuts	5 nuts	0.1 mg
Salmon, baked or broiled	3 ounces	0.2 mg
Sardines	3 ounces	0.3 mg
Crab	3 ounces	0.2 mg
Chicken	3 ounces	0.2mg
Mushrooms	3 ounces	0.4 mg
Broccoli	3 ounces	0.2 mg
Spinach, raw	1 cup	0.42 mg
Bread, whole wheat	1 slice	0.06 mg
Prunes	8	0.2 mg
Apricots, dried	1 ounce	0.2 mg
Avocado	1/2	0.1 mg

BEST FOOD SOURCES OF FOLATE INCLUDE:

Food	Serving Size	Amount of Folate
Calves' liver, braised	4 ounces	860.70 mcg
Lentils, cooked	1 cup	357.98 mcg
Spinach, boiled 1 minute	1 cup	262.80 mcg
Asparagus, boiled 1 minute	1 cup	262.80 mcg
Navy beans, cooked	1 cup	254.80 mcg
Pinto beans, cooked		294.12 mcg
Chickpeas (garbanzos), cooked	1 cup	282.08 mcg
Black beans, cooked	1 cup	255.94 mcg
Collard greens, steamed	1 cup	176.70 mcg
Turnip greens, cooked	1 cup	170.50 mcg
Lima beans, cooked	1 cup	156.23 mcg
Romaine lettuce	2 cups	151.98 mcg
Beets, cooked	1 cup	136.00 mcg
Split peas, cooked	1 cup	127.20 mcg
Papaya	1	115.52 mcg
Brussels sprouts, steamed	1 cup	93.60 mcg
Avocado slices	1 cup	90.37 mcg
Peanuts	1/4 cup	87.53 mcg
Sunflower seeds	1/4 cup	81.86 mcg
Winter squash, baked	1 cup	57.40 mcg
Cauliflower, steamed	1 cup	54.56 mcg

Food	Serving Size	Amount of Folate
Green beans, steamed	1 cup	41.63 mcg
Oranges	1	39.69 mcg
Summer squash, cooked slices	1 cup	36.18 mcg
Celery, raw	1 cup	33.6 mcg
Bell pepper, raw slices	1 cup	20.24 mcg
Carrots, raw	1 cup	17.08 mcg

As these tables show, simply enjoying one meal that includes a large tossed salad (leafy greens plus some favorite vegetables, such as carrots, celery, bell pepper, broccoli, cauliflower, beets, or green beans), along with 4 ounces of fish or a cup of beans, and snacking on a handful of peanuts, sunflower seeds, and/or an orange, a banana, or some papaya, can help meet your bones' vitamin B needs.

"C" Your Way to Stronger Bones

Vitamin C stimulates the activity of akaline phosphatase, an enzyme that is a marker for the formation of the bone-building osteoblasts; is necessary for the formation and secretion of osteoid, a cartilage-like material into which the osteoblasts deposit calcium; and is also required for the cross-linking of collagen fibrils in bone, which helps to form a strong bone matrix. Not getting enough vitamin C means not enough bone-building cells or docking stations for calcium inside your bones.[83]

A number of recent studies have confirmed vitamin C's importance for bone health. Researchers analyzing seventeen years of follow up data from the Framingham Osteoporosis Study noted that study participants whose diets provided the most vitamin C had significantly fewer hip and other fractures compared to those whose diets provided the lowest amounts of vitamin C.[84] A study carried out at the Hospital of Jaén, in Spain, confirmed this. This study involved 167 people aged 65 or older who had had a fragility fracture (a fracture that occurs during normal daily activities as a result of having weak, thin bones) plus 167 healthy controls of comparable age and sex. When study participants' diet was assessed for vitamin C intake, and their blood levels of vitamin C were measured, those whose diets provided the most vitamin C (and thus those whose blood levels of vitamin C were highest) were found to have a 69% lower risk of fracture! [85]

In another recent study, this one conducted in Australia, researchers randomly selected 533 nonsmoking women and checked their blood levels of a key biochemical marker of bone breakdown called C-telopeptide (CTx). Not only was CTx much lower in women taking supplemental vitamin C, but the longer the women had been taking vitamin C, the lower their CTx level.[86]

Many Americans are consuming far too little vitamin C to maintain healthy bones. In the third National Health and Nutrition Examination Survey (NHANES III, 1988–1994), approximately 13% of the US population was vitamin C deficient (blood levels lower than 11.4 micromols per liter). The most recent NHANES (2003–2004) showed some improvement, finding frank vitamin C deficiency in 7.1% of Americans.

However, there is a big difference between outright vitamin C deficiency—we're talking so little vitamin C that these folks were at risk for scurvy—and having enough of this nutrient available in your body to promote strong, healthy bones![87] Although the RDA for vitamin C was recently increased to 75 mg per day in women and 90 mg per day in men, this recommendation is still based on how much vitamin C is needed to prevent frank deficiency (think scurvy), not how much is needed to promote optimal health. In the medical research, intakes of vitamin C much higher than the RDAs have been related to better bone health. In postmenopausal women, greater bone mineral density was reported as vitamin C intake from supplements increased from 0 to 500 to 1,000 mg per day.[88]

FOODS RICH IN VITAMIN C

Food	Serving Size	Amount of Vitamin C
Papaya	1	187.87 mg
Bell pepper, red, raw, slices	1 cup	174.8 mg
Broccoli, steamed	1 cup	123.40 mg
Brussels sprouts	1 cup	96.72 mg
Strawberries	1 cup	81.65 mg
Oranges	1	69.69 mg
Cantaloupe	1 cup	67.52 mg
Kiwifruit	1	57.00 mg

In addition, vitamin C plays many vital roles in our white (immune) blood cells and is therefore rapidly depleted when we are ill, when we consume foods or beverages high in sugar, or when we are exposed to cigarette smoke.[89] Vitamin C levels are one-third lower in smokers compared to nonsmokers.[90] All these circumstances greatly increase our needs for vitamin C.

Pull out your trusty food diary and see how much vitamin C your diet is giving you each day.

CHAPTER 4

What Else Increases My Risk for Osteoporosis?

Osteoporosis, a Family Affair?

THE LEVEL OF PEAK BONE MINERAL DENSITY OR bone mass, which our bodies attain between 20 and 30 years of age, is greatly influenced by genetic factors.[91] Some studies suggest that up to 80% of how much peak bone mass each of us achieves is related to genetic factors! Young daughters of women with osteoporotic fractures have lower bone mass compared with other children their age, and *first-degree relatives* (the parents, brothers, sisters, or children) of women with osteoporosis tend to have lower bone mass than do first-degree relatives of women who do not have a family history of osteoporosis.[92]

The rate at which we lose bone after menopause is also impacted by our genetic inheritance. Although the genetic impact on the rate at which bone is lost with aging are less dramatic than our genes' effects on how much peak bone mass we achieve, our genes may still account for up to 56% of the variation in the rate at which bone loss occurs among different individuals.[93]

So, What Does This Mean for YOU?

Just as some people can smoke for 50 years and never develop lung cancer or COPD (chronic obstructive pulmonary disease), some people have an inborn ability to build and keep very strong, dense bones. If your mother, aunt, and/ or grandmother experienced a broken hip or other fragility fracture, however, chances are that you are not one of them!

This does *not* mean you are doomed to develop osteoporosis. You absolutely can be the first woman in your family in generations to go through your entire life with the beautiful, erect posture that comes from strong, healthy bones. But you will need to make the diet, lifestyle, and supplement choices outlined in this book that optimize bone health. Your bones need all the help you can provide.

Gastric Bypass: Free Pass? Not for Your Bones

Gastric bypass (or small-bowel resection) reduces the amount of absorptive surface area in the intestines, and by doing so lessens the body's ability to absorb not just fat and calories, but also all the nutrients needed to maintain and form healthy bone.

The gastric bypass (the medical term for it is the Roux-en-Y procedure) is the leading surgery to treat morbid obesity performed in the

United States. Since this operation causes the primary sites where calcium absorption occurs to be bypassed, patients become deficient in calcium and vitamin D. In response to these deficiencies, the body up-regulates the secretion and activity of parathyroid hormone. Parathyroid hormone has two bone-related effects: it causes an increase in the production of the most active form of vitamin D (1,25-dihydroxyvitamin D), which helps us absorb more calcium from food, but it also causes increased bone resorption (bone breakdown) to liberate more calcium for calcium's many other uses in the body.[94]

Calcium wears a lot of "hats" in the body, playing vital roles in a number of critical physiological processes not related to its use in bone. These include helping blood to clot, so we don't bleed to death when cut; helping nerves to send impulses and muscles to contract (in the case of the heart muscle, contraction = heartbeat); and regulating our cell membranes, so our cells can allow entry of what they need and send out what they don't.

Because these activities are essential to life, the body tightly controls the amount of calcium in the blood to ensure that sufficient calcium is available for them. Our bones, where approximately 99% of the calcium in our bodies is stashed, serve as a calcium "bank" from which withdrawals can be made to maintain normal blood concentrations whenever the need arises—which it surely will after gastric bypass (or if we fail to consume calcium-rich foods and/or supplemental calcium sufficient to meet our body's needs).

Gastric banding, another surgical procedure for morbid obesity, is a safer, potentially reversible, and effective alternative to the Roux-en-Y gastric bypass that has not been shown to produce as much bone loss as the Roux-en-Y procedure. In gastric banding, an inflatable silicone device is placed around the top portion of the stomach to create a small pouch at the top of the stomach that holds about 3.5 to 6.5 ounces of food. When a person eats, the pouch quickly fills with food, and the band slows its passage from the pouch to the lower part of the stomach. As soon as the upper part of the stomach registers as full, the brain is sent a message that the entire stomach is full, which helps the person eat smaller portions, eat less often, and lose weight over time. Within six to eight years, weight loss from gastric banding is comparable to that achieved by gastric bypass; however, many physicians and patients choose gastric bypass because it results in faster weight loss and resolution of diabetes.[95] The fact that some of the weight lost comes from the patient's bones is somehow overlooked.

What Does This Mean for YOU?

Either of these surgeries will lessen your body's ability to absorb calcium and the other nutrients necessary for bone health. If you have had or are considering either of these surgical interventions for morbid obesity, please discuss the potential adverse effects on your bones with your physician. Medical journal articles alerting physicians to these concerns are just beginning to appear, and many doctors remain unaware of these issues.[96]

Although increasing calcium or vitamin D intake does not suppress parathyroid hormone or prevent the acceleration in bone resorption caused by gastric bypass, it is possible that highly absorbable supplements may help lessen the damage.[97] Anyone who has had either of these surgeries should be using calcium supplements providing calcium citrate and not calcium carbonate.*

The Liver–Kidney Connection to Bone

You've probably heard something about how important vitamin D is for bone health. Here's why: vitamin D stimulates the absorption of calcium from the intestines and also calcium's resorption from the kidneys, greatly improving the likelihood that adequate calcium will be present in the bloodstream for all the body's calcium needs.

However, these effects of vitamin D do not occur until *after* vitamin D has been converted

---

* See page 57.

into its most active form in the body. This conversion occurs in two stages, the first of which takes place in the liver, and the second in the kidneys. For this reason, dysfunction in either the liver or the kidneys can compromise vitamin D activation, calcium absorption, and bone health.

Approximately 23% of patients with chronic liver disease have osteoporosis. You may be thinking that this couldn't possibly concern you, that liver disease is uncommon and caused only by alcoholism or hepatitis. You'd be wrong.

Today, the most rapidly increasing liver disease is nonalcoholic fatty liver disease or NAFLD, and it is caused by insulin resistance and type 2 diabetes. Following menopause, risk for NAFLD goes up significantly. In a surprising 55% of women over age 60, liver function is compromised by NAFLD.[98] High blood pressure and diabetes also increase risk for chronic kidney disease, which is estimated to affect 11.5% of adults aged 20 or older in the US.[99]

What Does This Mean for YOU?

NAFLD and other liver diseases often produce no noticeable symptoms and may therefore go undiagnosed. Particularly if you have been diagnosed with MetS (metabolic syndrome) or type 2 diabetes, be sure your annual physical includes the standard lab tests that check liver function.[100]

Symptoms of worsening kidney function are also unspecific and may go unnoticed. Symptoms include feeling generally unwell and loss of appetite. Check to be sure that the lab tests run for your annual physical include *creatinine*. Higher levels of creatinine indicate a decrease in kidney function and the ability to excrete waste products.

Anyone suffering from chronic liver or kidney disease is at significantly increased risk for vitamin D deficiency and osteoporosis. Supplemental vitamin D has been found to help lessen bone loss associated with liver and/or kidney disease.[101]

What's Hyperparathyroidism and Why Should My Bones Care?

Hyperparathyroidism is overactivity of the parathyroid glands (hyper = excessive, above normal), resulting in excessive production of parathyroid hormone. Hyperparathyroidism is divided into "primary" and "secondary" types.

"Primary" hyperparathyroidism is relatively rare. It's a disease of the parathyroid glands themselves, usually of unknown origin, and is almost always the more severe form. Sometimes surgery is required as part of treatment.

"Secondary" hyperparathyroidism is almost always milder, and not always diagnosed as such. Secondary hyperparathyroidism is not a disease (as the primary form is) but a protective response by the body to increase blood levels of calcium from unhealthy low levels caused by inadequate calcium intake or the many other causes listed below.

But, although parathyroid hormone causes an increase in the body's production of the most active form of vitamin D (1,25-dihydroxyvitamin D), which helps us absorb more calcium from our intestines, parathyroid hormone also causes increased osteoclast activity and bone resorption (bone breakdown) in order to liberate calcium from bone for calcium's many other immediate uses in the body.

Blood levels of calcium low enough to cause secondary hyperparathyroidism are typically due to not getting enough daily calcium, vitamin D deficiency, chronic kidney disease, chronic liver disease, low levels of stomach acid (hypochlorhydria, relatively common after age 50), malabsorption of calcium (and other minerals, most often caused by "hidden" gluten sensitivity), or gastric bypass surgery. Obesity has also been shown to increase parathyroid hormone levels, which, in addition, tend to increase with age in both men and women.

Above normal levels of parathyroid hormone have recently been associated not only with osteoporosis, but also with cognitive decline and senile dementia (Alzheimer's disease). The connection is most likely explained by the fact that sustained high levels of parathyroid hormone in the brain increase risk of calcium overloading, which leads to impaired blood flow and brain degeneration.[102]

Fortunately, a recent study involving 37 institutionalized women, ranging in age from their late 70s to late 80s, has shown that consumption of a fortified dairy product, containing only about 17–25% of the recommended daily intakes for calcium and vitamin D, lowered levels of parathyroid hormone and increased levels of both vitamin D and markers of bone formation in just one month.[103]

What Does This Mean for YOU?

The lab tests ordered at your annual physical should include blood levels of parathyroid hormone. Normal values range from 10–55 picograms per milliliter (pg/ml); however, recent research suggests values higher than 30 may indicate suboptimal intake of calcium and vitamin D.[104]

Higher than normal levels of parathyroid hormone indicate that you are not meeting your body's needs for calcium and vitamin D, and that you are at increased risk not only for osteo-porosis but cognitive decline and Alzheimer's disease. Work with your doctor to increase your consumption of calcium and vitamin D, and recheck your levels of parathyroid hormone after a month to two months on your new and improved bone health promotion program.

Is Your Thyroid on Overdrive?

Hyperthyroidism (a "hyperactive" thyroid) is a well-known risk factor for osteoporosis, regard-less of sex or age. The hormones produced and secreted by the thyroid gland regulate the body's metabolic rate. When thyroid hormone levels are too high, regardless of whether we are pre- or post-menopausal, female or male, it's like put-ting the body into overdrive, accelerating all its metabolic activities, including the rate at which bones are remodeled, all the time.

Each bone remodeling cycle involves 3–5 weeks of bone breakdown by osteoclasts followed by about 3 months during which osteoblasts lay down new bone to replace the bone that was removed. The result of the fast-forward bone metabolism seen in hyperthyroidism is increased bone resorption that leads to a loss of approximately 10% of bone mass per remodeling cycle. Not surprisingly, this can quickly result in lowered bone mineral density and increased risk of fracture.[105] Fortunately, hyperthyroidism is relatively uncommon.

Do Your Favorite Activities All Involve Sitting?

If you want to keep your bones, get moving! Exercise helps build and maintain bone mass by stimulating osteoblasts. It's true that younger individuals get more bone-building bang-for-their-exercise-buck—a 2–5% increase in bone mineral density (BMD) per year—but us older folks can still expect regular exercise to deliver a net gain in BMD of 1–3% per year.[106]

In contrast, if most of your day involves sitting, your sedentary lifestyle is rapidly and dramatically accelerating the loss of your bones. Numerous studies have confirmed this.[107] In one of the most recent, researchers studied 59 post-menopausal women with osteoporosis or osteopenia, 30 of whom followed a weight resistance exercise program for one year while the remaining 29 did not exercise. At the end of the study, the exercising women showed a 1.17% *increase* in BMD in the lumbar spine. The sedentary women *lost* 2.26% in their lumbar spine BMD.[108]

Aerobics, weight bearing, and resistance exercises have all been shown to be effective in increasing the bone mineral density of the spine in postmenopausal women, and walking is especially effective for building bone in the hips.[109]

Just walking briskly for 15 to 20 minutes a day can be the deciding factor in whether you lose or gain bone mass. In another recent study involving 37 sedentary women, 20 women remained sedentary while 17 took up brisk walking for an average of just 16.9 minutes each day. In the same study, in a second group of 31 women, 15 women who had been walking regularly for 1 year returned to their former sedentary lifestyle, while the remaining 16 women continued their brisk walking for a second year.

These 16 women walked an average of 20.8 minutes daily—an amount of time you could clock in during your lunch hour. By the end of the study, BMD, measured in the *calcaneus* (anklebone) had decreased significantly (by 2.7%) in the women who stopped walking and returned to a sedentary lifestyle, but increased significantly (7.4%) in the women who had been sedentary but changed their lifestyle to include a daily brisk walk.[110]

Even if you already have been diagnosed with osteopenia or osteoporosis, exercise can be a huge help in restoring the health of your bones. In another recent study, researchers looked at the effects of a group exercise program on BMD, pain, and quality of life in postmenopausal women with osteoporosis (16 women, average age 55.2 years) and osteopenia (17 women, average age 55.4 years). Each group followed the same group exercise program. For one hour three times a week for 21 weeks, all the women did a series of breathing, warm-up, stretching, strengthening, balance, stabilization, and cooling exercises. After the 21-week program, both groups showed significant improvements in their DEXA-score (DEXA is the gold standard x-ray procedure used to evaluate bone density*), pain score, BMD, and all the parameters of the Quality of Life Questionnaire of the European Foundation for Osteoporosis. Following the exercise program, 43.8% of the osteoporotic women had a DEXA-score that now showed only osteopenia, and 23.5% of the osteopenic women had a DEXA-score falling within the normal range![111]

Getting Any . . . Sunshine?

Are your bones getting their daily dose of sunshine vitamin? Sunshine begins your body's bone-building process. Sunlight on exposed, *sunscreen-free* skin changes a compound in the skin called 7-dehydrocholesterol into vitamin D_3 (cholecalciferol). (Sunscreen SPF 8 reduces sunlight's ability to trigger the conversion of 7-dehydrocholesterol into vitamin D_3 by 95%.) This is the first of the three steps through which your

---

* See page 125.

body activates vitamin D into the form in which it is able to stimulate the absorption of calcium.

You don't have to spend hours being unprotected from the sun's skin-wrinkling rays or possibly increasing your risk for skin cancer. In the summer, all you need is 20–30 minutes of sun exposure, during which time, as much as 10,000 IU of vitamin D can be produced in our skin.

Once awakened by the kiss of sunlight on your skin, cholecalciferol is transported to the liver and converted into 25-hydroxycholecalciferol [25(OH)D$_3$], a compound five times as potent as cholecalciferol. 25-hydroxycholecalciferol is then sent to the kidneys where it is converted into 1,25-dihydroxycholecalciferol [1,25(OH)D$_3$], which is 10 times as potent as cholecalciferol and the most active form of vitamin D in the body.*

If you live north of 35° latitude (i.e., in any of the states north of North Carolina, Tennessee, Arkansas, Oklahoma, New Mexico, or Arizona, or in the northern part of California, or in Oregon

---

* You can see why liver or kidney problems can cause bone loss. For more on this, see page 87.

or Washington state), you are at increased risk for vitamin D deficiency. Why? Because the wavelength in sunlight needed to produce vitamin D in the skin (UVB radiation of 290 to 320 nm) is not available in these areas during the winter months and possibly for even more of the year.

In addition to people living in northern latitudes, individuals whose sun exposure is limited are at significant risk for vitamin D deficiency.[112] This would include those who are homebound or work in occupations that keep them indoors, preventing exposure to sunlight; wear clothing that completely covers the body (we knew wearing a burqa would not only keep us off the Best Dressed List, but is physically bad for us);[113] or always use sunscreen.

Even if you live in a sunny climate, sun exposure alone may not produce blood levels of vitamin D adequate for bone (and overall) health. Your vitamin D levels (as measured by the serum 25-hydroxyvitamin D test) should be at the very least 30 nanograms per milliliter (ng/ml) or 75 nanomoles per liter (nmol/L, an alternate measurement that is often used). Many physicians now recommend that 25-hydroxyvitamin D levels be between 60 and 100 ng/ml, the so-called "tropical optimum." But even in Hawaii, one recent 3-month study found that only half of the healthy and racially diverse young adult participants, whose average sun exposure was 29 hours each week, achieved blood levels of vitamin D of 30 ng/ml (75 nmol/L).[114]

If you are deficient in vitamin D, you will not absorb calcium effectively. Without adequate vitamin D, the intestine absorbs only 10–15% of the dietary or supplemental calcium you consume.[115]

Many studies have documented the key role vitamin D plays in bone health. Most of the research has been done using both calcium and vitamin D, but even a study using vitamin D_3 alone found that supplementation with 700 IU/day reduced the rate of hip fracture in elderly women (average age 84) by nearly 60%—from 1.3% to 0.5%.[116]

In another study of 3,270 healthy women, whose average age was again 84, for 18 months, half the women were given 800 mg of vitamin D along with 1,200 mg of calcium daily, while the other half received a placebo. Among those treated with vitamin D and calcium, the number of hip fractures was 43% lower and the number of nonvertebral fractures was 32% lower compared to those given the placebo. BMD in the femur (thigh bone) increased 2.7% in the women taking vitamin D and calcium, while decreasing 4.6% in the placebo group.[117]

Other large studies have confirmed these results, including a 2-year, multicenter study involving 583 institutionalized women whose average age was 85 years. In the women given vitamin D_3 (800 mg) along with calcium (1,200 mg) daily, parathyroid hormone levels returned to normal within 6 months (one of the effects of too little vitamin D is increased levels of parathyroid hormone, which causes increased osteoclast activity and bone breakdown*). In the women receiving vitamin D and calcium, BMD remained stable, while decreasing 2.36% in the women receiving the placebo.[118]

---

* See page 83.

The bone-health bottom line here is: you should consider a vitamin D_3 supplement. In healthy adults who regularly avoid sunlight exposure or always use sunscreen (like most of us wrinkle-avoiding women), a review of the research by the Vitamin D Council (www.vitamindcouncil.org), a nonprofit organization whose directors are among the world's leading experts on vitamin D, indicates a necessity to supplement with 2,000 to 5,000 IU of vitamin D daily. [119]

According to the Vitamin D Council, you can ensure your vitamin D levels are adequate for bone health by:

Regularly getting outside to enjoy a half hour of midday sun exposure in the late spring, summer, and early fall, exposing as much of your skin as possible (but being careful not to get a sunburn). Then you can apply sunscreen and don a hat.

Taking 5,000 IU of vitamin D_3 per day for 2–3 months, then getting a blood test run to check your levels of 25-hydroxyvitamin D_3. Work with your doctor to adjust your dosage of supplemental vitamin D so your blood levels are *at least* 30 ng/ml (75 nmol/L). A number of medical experts involved in vitamin D research now feel that optimal blood levels of vitamin D should run between 50–80 ng/ml (or 125–200 nmol/L) year-round.

Gloria Vanderbilt Once Said, "A Woman Can't Be Too Rich or Too Thin." She Was Half-Wrong.

Anorexia nervosa, an eating disorder character-ized by intense fear of gaining weight and becom-ing fat, despite being underweight (weighing less than 85% of the weight considered normal or healthy for one's height and build), causes bone loss, particularly in the spine and hip.[120] This is not surprising since bones cannot be built with-out a whole team of nutrients and also respond by strengthening when stressed by weight— which is why resistance exercises help build bone.

Heavier women put some stress on their bones just by walking around; thin women don't. But this is not a recommendation to become obese. Being overweight promotes inflammation and is much more harmful than helpful to your bones. Stress your bones by exercising, and not only will you build bone, you'll fit into your skinny jeans.

Avoiding food, self-induced vomiting, use of laxatives, diuretics, and/or appetite suppressants is a sure-fire recipe for bone starvation. Lack of sufficient nourishment not only causes a pre-menopausal woman to stop menstruating and lose bone, but also causes her to lose muscle and turn into a Skeletor cartoon character look-alike.

The stress that muscles put on bone when they contract is a key "time to build more bone" signal. Women are already at a bone-building disadvantage compared to men because our muscles are smaller. Cannibalize your muscles, and you thin your bones. The complete loss of menstrual periods, *amenorrhea*, occurs largely because the body is no longer willing to use the energy needed to produce estrogen, which as mentioned earlier,* regulates osteoclasts, preventing them from removing too much bone. Maybe you should stop reading now and go get a healthy, calcium-rich snack?

------

* See page 4.

Bone-Busting Patent Medicines

If you are taking any of the following patent medicines, work with your physician to help compensate for their bone-destroying effects or, if possible, to find an alternative less harmful to your bones.

Avandia® (rosiglitazone) and Actos® (pioglitazone): Use of the diabetes patent medicines Avandia® or Actos® for more than a year doubles to triples risk of hip fractures.[121]

These patent medicines, members of a class of patent medicines called thiazolidinediones (also known as glitazones), are insulin-sensitizing medications that account for approximately 21% of the oral blood sugar-lowering patent medicines used in the US. Although their main therapeutic effects occur in fat tissue, muscles, and the liver, studies show they affect bone as well. They do so by triggering mesenchymal stem cells, which can become any one of several different types of cells, including osteoblasts, chondrocytes (cells that produce cartilage), or adipocytes (fat cells), into choosing to become

adipocytes. When you take these patent medicines, your body makes more fat and less bone.

Because studies have demonstrated accelerated
bone loss, impaired bone mineral density, and
increased fracture risk for thiazolidinedione users,
clinicians have been told to carefully assess the
fracture risk in their patients with type 2 diabetes
before starting them on thiazolidinediones.[122]

Anticonvulsants: Barbituates such as phe-
nobarbital or Mysoline (primidone), alter the
metabolism of vitamin D. Dilantin (phenytoin)
interferes with vitamin D and may also cause a
deficiency of folate or B_6, or a reduction in blood
levels of vitamin K, all of which are essential for
building and maintaining bone.

Chronic Opioid Therapy: Used in the management of chronic pain, opioid patent medicines
(e.g., morphine, codeine, hydrocodone, oxyco-
done, methadone, tramadol) greatly impact the
production of a number of hormones, including two with significant effects on bone: estrogen and thyroid stimulating hormone (TSH). A
study of 47 women, aged 30 to 75, who were

using oral or transdermal opioids for control of nonmalignant pain found estradiol levels were 57% lower than in control subjects! These patent medicines inhibit estrogen production so effectively that among premenopausal women, menstruation typically ceases soon after initiating opioid therapy. In contrast, opioid patent medicines *increase* the production of TSH, which directly suppresses bone remodeling. The combined effect of suppressing estrogen production and increasing that of TSH is greatly increased risk of osteoporosis. Women needing opioids for relief of chronic pain should discuss bioidentical hormone replacement with their physicians.[123]

Glucocorticoid patent medicines: Often mistakenly termed "cortisone," these patent medicines include Prednisone, Prednisolone, Kenalog, Dexamethasone, and nearly anything else ending in "-one," along with the nonpatentable Cortef, which is bioidentical cortisol, but as a prescription often used in excess of normal body levels. These patent medicines kill osteocytes (which is what osteoblasts turn into after they begin secreting the bone matrix). Thus, these patent medicines cause a rapid weakening of bone architecture (within 6 months of initiating treatment) even at very low doses. In addition, the glucocorticoid patent medicines deplete the body of vitamin D_3, interfering with normal calcium metabolism and absorption. One reason smoking is so harmful to bone is that nicotine causes the body to produce excess cortisol.[124]

Antacids/Proton-pump inhibitors: For calcium to be absorbed, it must first be made soluble and ionized by stomach acid. These patent medicines inhibit or even totally prevent your body's ability to produce stomach acid.*

Are Your Bones Going Up in Smoke?

Smokers lose bone more rapidly, have lower bone mass (a full one-third of a standard deviation less at the hip and a one-tenth standard deviation less for all sites combined), and a

---

* For a full discussion on this, please see "I Need Stomach Acid to Absorb Calcium?," page 55.

higher fracture rate. In addition, women who smoke reach menopause, when estrogen levels plummet causing bone loss, up to two years earlier than their nonsmoking peers.[125]

Approximately 19% of the hip fractures occurring in a study that pooled data from three population studies involving a total of 13,393 women and 17,379 men were attributable to smoking.[126] In other research, smoking increased risk of spinal osteoporosis in men by 230%![127]

Why Is Smoking So Harmful to Your Bones? Two Key Reasons: Cadmium and Nicotine.

CADMIUM

Cadmium, a toxic metal that is present in the environment both naturally and as a pollutant from industrial and agricultural sources, stimulates the formation and activity of osteoclasts, the cells that break down bone.[128] Cadmium also inhibits the normal inactivation of cortisol. While cortisol is an essential-to-life hormone, excess amounts of cortisol are known to contribute to osteoporosis and hypertension, as well as other problems. The two main sources of exposure to cadmium in the general population are tobacco smoking and food grown in areas in which the soil or coastline waters are contaminated with high levels of cadmium.

Cigarettes are loaded with cadmium. About 10% of the cadmium they contain is inhaled through smoking, and since cadmium is much more effectively absorbed through the lungs than the gut, as much as 50% of the cadmium inhaled via cigarette smoke may be absorbed. Smokers typically have 4–5 times higher blood concentrations and 2–3 times higher kidney concentrations of cadmium.[129]

Cadmium gets into the food supply in foods harvested from cadmium-polluted areas, including shellfish (oysters, mussels, etc.[130]); vegetable, grain, and fruit crops; and meat and dairy products derived from animals pastured in areas with high levels of cadmium in the soils.[131] In general, cadmium concentrations in urban areas tend to be higher than in rural areas of the United States.[132] In areas with high soil levels of cadmium, house dust can also be an important route of exposure.[133]

The use of cadmium to stabilize plastic, as a red and yellow pigment, and in corrosion-resistant coating for steel and copper alloys has declined, but this toxic metal is still widely used in batteries, predominantly rechargeable nickel-cadmium (Ni-Cd) batteries, and in cadmium telluride solar panels. Cadmium may also be present in children's jewelry imported from China. In 2010, a US Consumer Product Safety Commission investigation found 12% of the 103 such items tested from New York, Ohio, Texas, and California contained at least 10% cadmium; one of the items tested contained 91% cadmium.[134]

Classified as a carcinogen, cadmium accumulates in the human body, has a half-life for elimination ranging from 20 to 40 *years*, and is mainly stored in the liver and kidneys. Cadmium causes kidney dysfunction, kidney stone formation, osteomalacia (bone pain), and osteoporosis.[135] (Remember our earlier discussion* of how

---

* See page 87.

vitamin D is activated in the liver and kidneys into the form in which it helps the body absorb calcium? Cadmium can really mess this up.)

Analysis of NHANES (National Health and Nutrition Examination Survey) data indicates that women 50 years of age or older with urinary cadmium levels between 0.50 and 1.00 microgram/gram creatinine* had a 43% greater risk for hip-BMD-defined osteoporosis, compared to women with urinary cadmium levels less than 0.50 microg/g.

You can minimize your exposure to cadmium by not smoking or hanging out with people who do; avoiding consumption of oysters, scallops, and shellfish from coastal areas along the New England states and Great Lakes with high

---

* Creatinine is used as a marker since it is excreted at basically the same rate by everyone, while the amount of urine we produce can vary greatly from person to person. For this reason, the amount of creatinine present in a urine sample is used as a means of standardizing kidney output of other compounds in the urine, such as, in this case, cadmium. Seventy-three percent of US women aged 50 or older are estimated to have cadmium body burdens of greater than 0.50 micrograms/gram creatinine. These results suggest that 31% of the osteoporosis prevalence among American women at least 50 years old may be attributable to cadmium![136]

cadmium levels; dusting regularly and using a HEPA air filter to improve the air quality in your home and office.

NICOTINE

Nicotine, even in low concentrations, depresses osteoblast activity. Levels of osteocalcin—a protein secreted by osteoblasts that plays a key role in depositing calcium in bone—are much lower in smokers.[137] If you smoke to keep your weight down, you'll be interested to know that osteocalcin also plays important roles in promoting insulin secretion and insulin sensitivity. Insulin is the hormone that gets sugars inside your cells where they can be burned for energy instead of stored as fat. Lack of sensitivity to insulin promotes weight gain and is a key factor in metabolic syndrome, type 2 diabetes, and obesity. Thus, smoking thins your bones while expanding your waistline.[138]

In concentrations typically seen in heavy smokers, nicotine is toxic to osteoblasts.[139] Nicotine also increases the rate at which the liver clears estrogen from the body, and thus, in postmenopausal women, can completely cancel out the benefits of oral estrogen replacement, not only on bone health, but on hot flashes, vaginal thinning and dryness, and cholesterol.[140]

Data from the Third National Health and Nutrition Examination Survey, which included 14,060 subjects, found that blood levels of cotinine, a metabolite of nicotine and marker for exposure to cigarette smoke (whether active or passive), were inversely related to BMD in both men and women. More nicotine exposure = less bone.[141]

The good news for smokers: if you quit, you will quickly regain your ability to build bone. When postmenopausal women who smoked at least ten cigarettes a day were randomly assigned to a 4-month smoking cessation program, and were then followed for an additional year, the women who quit smoking quickly began rebuilding bone and gained 2.9% in BMD in their femoral trochanter (top of the thigh bone) and 1.52% in their hips.[142]

More than Two Drinks of Liquor Makes Bone Loss Much Quicker

Alcohol has a dose-dependent toxic effect on osteoblast activity. One to two drinks a day appears to be beneficial. More than two drinks a day prevents bone repair and renewal, and significantly increases fracture risk.[143]

Using data from the Third National Health and Nutrition Examination Survey, researchers found that moderate drinkers (less than 29 drinks per month) actually had higher BMD than abstainers. Moderate consumption of alcohol translated to 2.1% higher BMD in men and 3.8% higher BMD in postmenopausal women.[144] Another large study, this one involving 11,032 women and 5,939 men, found no increase in fracture risk when two ounces or less of alcohol was consumed daily, but drinking more than this increased risk of any osteoporotic fracture by 38% and hip fracture by 68%.[145]

Your choice of which alcoholic beverage to consume can also affect the health of your bones. Several recent studies suggest moderate intake (no more than two servings a day) of beer and/or wine may have beneficial effects on bone. (One serving of beer = 8 ounces; one serving of wine = 4 ounces.) A study of 1,697 healthy women, of whom 710 were premenopausal, 176 were perimenopausal, and 811 were postmenopausal, found that beer drinkers had slightly higher bone mass.[146]

A second large study involving 1,182 men, 1,289 postmenopausal woman, and 248 premenopausal women found bone mineral density was 3.0–4.5% greater in men consuming 2 daily drinks of alcohol or beer, and 5.0–8.3 greater in postmenopausal women consuming 1–2 drinks of alcohol or wine daily. More than 2 drinks a day, however, was associated with significantly lower (3.0–5.2% lower) bone mineral density in the hip and spine in men.

Beer's beneficial effects on bone are thought to be due to its silicon content. One can of beer contains around 7 milligrams of silicon; a 4-ounce glass of wine provides around 1 milligram of silicon. (For comparison, a half cup of cooked spinach contains around 5 milligrams of silicon.)

Wine's bone benefits may be linked to its content of phytochemicals, especially the resveratrol present in red wine, which has been shown to have estrogenic effects and might therefore help protect against bone loss in postmenopausal women in whom estrogen levels are low. In rat studies, resveratrol has been shown to have an estrogenic effect and to promote increased BMD in ovariectomized rats (rats whose ovaries have been removed to simulate menopause).[147]

CHAPTER 5

What Men Don't Know Can Increase Their Risk for Osteoporosis

THE SAME FACTORS THAT AFFECT BONE HEALTH IN women also affect men's bones, although in men, peak bone mass is greater and the decline in male hormones (androgens) occurs somewhat later and is not as rapid. Despite these protective factors, approximately 25% of men will have an osteoporotic fracture during their lifetime, and men account for 30% of hip and 20% of vertebral fragility fractures.

More men will experience an osteoporotic fracture than will have a heart attack or stroke, or will develop Alzheimer's disease, prostate cancer, or lung cancer. The incidence of osteoporosis-related fracture in men exceeds that of lung and prostate cancer combined![148]

What Are the Key Risk Factors for Osteoporosis in Men?

- Bone-busting patent medicines (see Chapter 2, beginning on page 11).
- Vitamin D deficiency: A number of recent surveys indicate less than 1/3 of white males and less than 1/10 of black males have optimal vitamin D status.[149] One of the latest, the MrOS study, recently found 72% of men were deficient in vitamin D.[150]
- Hyperthyroidism (see page 90).
- Increased parathyroid hormone levels (see page 91).
- Excessive alcohol consumption (see page 115) for men, it's "more than 2 drinks of liquor, and bone loss is quicker."

- Smoking (see pages 108–114).
- Gastrointestinal disease: not only do the pro-inflammatory compounds produced by the body in conditions such as Irritable Bowel Syndrome and Crohn's Disease promote disturbances in bone and mineral metabolism,[151] but the patent medicines used to suppress symptoms (e.g., corticosteroids, stomach acid blockers) prevent healthy bone remodeling.[152]
- Osteoarthritis: inflammation activates osteoclasts and promotes bone less.[153]
- *Andropause*: lack of testosterone results in insufficient production of estrogen to maintain bone (see page 54).[154]
- *Sarcopenia* (loss of muscle mass with aging): the drop in male hormones that occurs with aging reduces not only muscle mass but bone mass, and is associated with an increase in fat mass. More than one-third of people over age 65 years fall annually and approximately 5% of falls lead to fracture.[155]
- Prostate cancer—androgen deprivation therapy (same reasoning as Andropause; see page 54).[156]

- Malabsorption of calcium and other minerals secondary to hypochlorhydria (low stomach acid) is more common in older men, especially those over 60.
- Malabsorption of calcium, other minerals, amino acids, and other nutrients secondary to "hidden" (no symptoms or minimal symptoms) gluten sensitivity. Osteoporosis or osteopenia (beginning bone loss) in men under 50 is frequently due to "hidden" gluten sensitivity, which is most accurately detected by testing for secretory IgA gluten antibodies in a stool specimen.

CHAPTER 6

Chances Are, You Are Already Losing Bone

I F YOU ARE CONSUMING THE STANDARD AMERICAN diet, not getting regular exercise, wear sunscreen all the time and/or get little sun exposure, you have lots of company. You are following the normal lifestyle of people living in the United States—and you are losing bone.

Americans' nutrient-poor diet, combined with pandemic vitamin D insufficiency and a couch-potato lifestyle is the perfect recipe for osteoporosis. Plus, because, initially, bone loss causes no symptoms, most people live under the illusion that even women don't lose much bone before menopause—an assumption that could not be further from the truth!

The only way to find out how your bones are doing is by N-telopeptide and DEXA Testing, So let's talk about this next.

How Can I Tell If I'm Losing Bone?

You're losing bone. The real question is how much, how quickly? Even in adults, normal healthy bone is dynamic, living tissue that is constantly being broken down (or *resorbed*) and rebuilt. In fact, up to 10% of all your bone mass is likely to be undergoing remodeling at any point in time. Normally, it's a balanced process in which bone rebuilding keeps pace with bone breakdown. In osteoporosis, however, bone resorption outpaces bone formation.

Actually, after age 40, it's normal for bone mass to decline up to 1.5% to 2% per year in men as well as in women, a small loss that should not seriously compromise bone strength. Women, however, are at high risk of losing a good deal more bone mass than men and developing osteoporosis because of their smaller size (smaller bones, smaller muscles) and the drop in female hormones, estrogen and progesterone, that occurs with menopause.

What Tests Are Used to Check for Bone Loss? What Qualifies as Osteoporosis?

The DEXA and N-telopeptide tests are the most widely used tests to evaluate bone mineral density and the rate at which bone is being lost.

In women, the World Health Organization defines *osteopenia* (bone thinning) as a bone mineral density between 1 and 2.5 *standard deviations** and osteoporosis as a bone mineral density 2.5 standard deviations below peak bone mass (the amount of bone mass that is

---

* Standard deviation is a statistical measurement that, in this case, shows how much the bone mass of a specific woman differs from that of the "average" healthy 20 year old woman, which is the time in a woman's life when her bone mass is highest.

normally seen in a 20 year old healthy female) as measured by *DEXA*.[157]

The *DEXA*—which stands for "dual energy X-ray absorptiometry"—is the most widely used and most thoroughly studied bone density measurement test. During a DEXA, two X-ray beams with differing energy levels are aimed at the patient's bones. The amount of the beams absorbed by soft tissue is subtracted, and the individual's BMD is then determined from the amount of the beams her bones have absorbed.)

The *N-telopeptide* test measures the rate of bone loss. Also written as NTx, this is a urine test, which measures the breakdown products of bone, such as the compound from which it gets its name: cross-linked N-telopeptide of type I collagen. By measuring the amount of this compound excreted in the urine, the NTx measures how quickly bone is breaking down. (Pyrilinks-D is another test for bone loss, but much less often used at present.)

The DEXA test is best used to measure bone density, while Ntx urinary bone resorption assessments are used to measure the rate of bone loss and are thus helpful for monitoring the success (or failure) of therapy. The NTx test provides much quicker feedback than the DEXA, which can take up to two years to detect a therapeutic response. Unfortunately, even though the NTx (and Pyrilinks-D) tests measure the bone loss side of the everyday, this is only one side of the dynamic "bone-building / bone loss" equation. At present, there is no widely available test for the degree of everyday bone-building.

Additional tests may be used to determine potential causes of bone loss. These include gastric acid levels, serum calcium, 24-hour urinary calcium, parathyroid hormone, thyroid stimulating hormone, free thyroxine (the T3 thyroid hormone) levels, serum albumin and serum alkaline phosphatase (which checks on liver function), and vitamin D levels.

What to Expect If You Don't Take Steps to Actively Prevent Bone Loss: What Are the Signs and Symptoms of Osteoporosis?

Initially, as bone thins, its loss rarely produces any symptoms—for which reason, osteoporosis has been called "the silent disease," but this is part of the problem! For many, the first symptom is a broken bone or an alarming DEXA test.

As the disease progresses, if symptoms occur, they can include:

- Backache
- Neck pain
- Muscle pain
- Bone tenderness

Late symptoms include:

- Severe backache in either the upper or lower regions of the back
- Loss of height
- Sudden back pain with a cracking sound indicating vertebral (spinal bone) fracture

- Fractures, especially of the hip, arm, or wrist, occurring during normal daily activity or with minor injury, such as slipping and falling
- Spinal deformities—a stooped posture or hunchback, resulting from loss of bone mass and/or from multiple vertebral compression fractures

PART 4

How to Have Strong Bones For Life

CHAPTER 7

Strong Bones for Life, Naturally

What Your Bones Really Need to Stay Strong

AS YOU NOW KNOW, BONE IS DYNAMIC, LIVING tissue that is constantly being broken down and rebuilt, regardless of one's age or sex. Until recently, not getting enough calcium and women's postmenopausal drop in estrogen were singled out as the only issues. Today, vitamin D's importance for bone health is once again being recognized.

It's true that calcium, vitamin D, and estrogen play key roles in preventing osteoporosis, but maintaining healthy bones throughout life requires a good deal more than simply calcium, estrogen, and vitamin D. Normal bone metabolism is a complex dance among over two dozen nutrients including the vitamins K (especially K_2), B_6, B_{12}, and folate as well as vitamin D, and the minerals boron, magnesium, phosphorous, zinc, manganese, copper, silicon, molybdenum, selenium—and possibly strontium—as well as calcium.

Also, while estrogen regulates the action of osteoclasts, specialized bone cells that remove dead portions of demineralized bone, progesterone is required by the osteoblasts, the bone-forming cells that pull calcium, magnesium, and phosphorous from the blood to build new bone mass.

What you need to know about each of these factors essential for building and maintaining healthy bones is discussed below.

Bone-Building Vitamins

VITAMIN D

What it Does

Vitamin D is essential for calcium's absorption from the intestines, and for its re-absorption from the kidneys (so it is not excreted in the urine), and therefore increases calcium's availability, while also stimulating its use in bone. Vitamin D deficiency leads not only to muscle weakness, which increases the risk of falling, but to osteopenia and osteoporosis—all three increase your risk of fracture.

In addition to its roles in calcium absorption, vitamin D is now known to affect genetic transcription—the process that directs our cells' DNA to turn on certain genes, which then send out messenger RNA to make certain proteins, while turning off other genes and preventing the production of other proteins. It's complicated, but what it boils down to is that not having enough vitamin D on board can result in a wide array of harmful outcomes, including not only osteoporosis, but also depression, many common cancers, autoimmune diseases like multiple sclerosis, susceptibility to infectious diseases, and cardiovascular diseases. Your entire body, not just your bones, needs vitamin D!

How Much Do I Need?

Most Americans are not getting anywhere near enough vitamin D. Current official recommendations for women aged 50 or older are only 600 IU per day, but leading vitamin D researchers and the majority of experts believe we need *at least* 1,000 IU per day. Many vitamin D experts are now recommending somewhere between 2,000 IU and 5,000 IU, or even as much as 10,000 IU, per day. Americans' average daily intake of vitamin D, which is found in small amounts in fortified milk and in fatty fish such as salmon and sardines, is only 200 IU![158]

To determine if you are vitamin D deficient— or more likely, how serious a vitamin D deficiency you have—it's best to have a blood test run to check your levels of 25-hydroxyvitamin

D_3 [you may also see this written as $25(OH)D_3$ or $25(OH)D$].

If your blood levels of vitamin D are not *at least* 30 ng/ml (or if the "nmol/L" measure is used, your blood levels should be 75 nmol/L), work with your doctor to fine tune your dosage of supplemental vitamin D that will, in 2–3 months, raise your blood levels to at least this amount.

Many medical experts involved in vitamin D research now feel that *optimal* blood levels of vitamin D should run between 50–80 ng/ml (or 125–200 nmol/L) year-round.[159] As mentioned earlier, the Vitamin D Council (www.vitamindcouncil.org), a nonprofit organization whose directors are among the foremost vitamin D experts in the world, recommends simply taking 5,000 IU of vitamin D daily for 2–3 months, then having your blood levels of vitamin D checked.*

---

* Please see "Getting Any . . . Sunshine?," page 97.

What to Look For in a Supplement

Supplemental vitamin D is available in two forms, ergocalciferol (D_2, a plant-derived form) and cholecalciferol (D_3, the form found in fatty fish, which is also the form that is produced naturally when the cholesterol in human skin cells is exposed to ultraviolet light). Both D_2 and D_3 are technically referred to as "provitamin D" since humans can convert both forms into the most active form of vitamin D, which is called calcitriol [$1,25(OH)_2D_3$]. (Remember, we do this via a two-step process that starts in the liver and is completed in the kidneys, so both organs need to be functioning properly.) However, D_3 is a better supplement choice than D_2 since D_3 is much more biologically active.

In humans, vitamin D_3 has been found to be two-and-a-half times more effective than vitamin D_2 in raising and maintaining blood levels of vitamin D, and D_3 also has a 40% greater ability to bind to the vitamin D receptor (VDR) on our cells, which is the way in which vitamin D exerts all its effects. [160]

Safety Issues

You may see misleading information about how much vitamin D is safe to take. The reason for the confusion is that the Upper Tolerable Intake Levels (ULs), which tell us how much of a nutrient we can take daily without risk of toxicity, were set for vitamin D by the National Academy of Sciences back in 1997. At that time, the UL for vitamin D intake in adults, including pregnant and breastfeeding women (for whom recommended nutrient intakes are often higher) was set at just 2,000 IU per day.

We now know that this UL is way too low. Clinical research has clearly shown that vitamin D supplementation in the range of 1,000–2,000 IU per day is not high enough to restore vitamin D health in most individuals with chronic vitamin D deficiency—and this means most Americans, since the vast majority of us are deficient in vitamin D.

If the UL for vitamin D that was set in 1997 were correct, we would all become vitamin D toxic every summer! Just being outside in the summer sunshine for an afternoon can provide an adult with an amount of vitamin D equivalent to taking 10,000 IU/day. And a significant body of clinical research has now shown that prolonged intake of 10,000 IU/day of vitamin D_3 is unlikely to cause any adverse effects in almost all individuals in the general population, which is the criterion used to set the UL.[161]

Although you are highly unlikely to see any adverse effects from taking vitamin D, it's best to know what the symptoms of too much vitamin D (vitamin D toxicity) are. These include loss of appetite, nausea, vomiting, high blood pressure, and kidney malfunction. In addition, individuals with *primary hyperparathyroidism* (an overactive parathyroid gland whose overactivity is not caused by vitamin D deficiency) are at increased risk for vitamin D toxicity and should not take supplemental vitamin D without consulting with a physician.

You should monitor your vitamin D status within 2–3 months of beginning to take supplemental vitamin D to ensure you are taking enough, but not more vitamin D than you need. Ask your doctor to re-order the lab test that checks your blood levels of $25(OH)D_3$. This is the major circulating form of vitamin D in the blood, and the form of the vitamin that is the true barometer of your vitamin D status. Adequate supplies of vitamin D are indicated by blood levels of $25(OH)D_3$ of *at least* 30 ng/ml (nanograms per milliliter) or 75 nmol/L (nanomoles per liter), depending upon which form of measurement, ng/ml or nmol/L, the lab running your blood test uses to report these results.

VITAMIN K

What It Does

Vitamin K plays a number of life-saving roles in our bodies, among which helping our blood to clot is the most critical. Without vitamin K, specifically, the K_1 form of this nutrient, we would bleed to death from even a tiny cut. In its K_2 form, vitamin K is responsible for ensuring that calcium is deposited in our bones—and not in our arteries!

Vitamin K_1 (*phylloquinone*), the type of vitamin K found in plants (phyllo = plant), especially leafy greens, can be converted by health-promoting bacteria in our intestines into vitamin

K_2 (*menaquinone*). Vitamin K_2 activates *osteocalcin*, the protein required for calcium to be deposited in bone. Once activated by K_2, osteocalcin can attract calcium molecules and anchor them into the hydroxyapatite crystals that form our bone matrix. K_2 also activates another protein called matrix-Gla protein, which prevents calcium from depositing in and "calcifying" soft tissue, such as our heart, arteries, breasts, or kidneys.

Vitamin K, in both its K_1 and K_2 forms, also greatly lessens the body's production of a wide range of proinflammatory compounds (including interleukin-6, tumor necrosis factor, and C-reactive protein) and, by doing so, lowers overall inflammation. This is important for bone health because when inflammation increases, this signals the body to also increase production and activation of osteoclasts, the cells that break down bone. Before menopause, estrogen puts a damper on women's production of proinflammatory compounds, but as estrogen levels drop with menopause, the body's production of proinflammatory molecules increases. Vitamin K is especially important for postmenopausal women since it helps keep inflammation, and therefore the production of osteoclasts, under control.[162]

Not eating lots of leafy greens (not supplying your body with plenty of vitamin K) results in impaired calcium deposition in bone (and increased likelihood of calcified arteries) because, without enough vitamin K around, neither osteocalcin, which puts calcium in bone, nor matrix-Gla protein, which keeps calcium out of soft tissues, can be activated.[163]

Although you probably haven't heard about it, vitamin K's importance for bone health has been known for a long time. For more than 20 years, human studies have demonstrated that vitamin K insufficiency increases risk of osteoporotic fracture. Research published in 1984 found that patients who suffered osteoporotic fractures had vitamin K levels 70% lower than age-matched controls, an association that has been repeatedly confirmed.[164] One trial involving almost 900 men and women found a 65% greater risk of hip fracture in those with the lowest blood levels of vitamin K compared to those with the highest levels of the nutrient, who averaged an intake of K_1 of 254 micrograms per day.[165]

Other human research has shown that vitamin K_2, specifically, is an effective treatment against osteoporosis, even in individuals taking corticosteroids, patent medicines well known to have the adverse side effect of greatly accelerating bone loss. Over a two-year period, the rate of vertebral fractures in patients taking corticosteroids who were also taking vitamin K_2 was 13.3% compared to 41% in the patients taking corticosteroids but no K_2.[166]

K_2 has also been shown to rebuild bone in patients with osteoporosis. In a 24-week study, 80 patients with osteoporosis were given either 90 milligrams per day of vitamin K_2 (the menaquinone-4 form)—don't worry, what this means is explained below—or placebo. In those taking K_2, bone mineral density (BMD) increased in the second metacarpal (the middle bone in the index finger) an average of 2.2%. In those given the placebo, BMD decreased an average of 7.31%.[167]

A review study that looked at the results of all randomized controlled human trials lasting at least 6 months that evaluated the use of vitamin K_1 or K_2 to lower fracture risk found 13 trials that met this criterion. All but one showed that both vitamin K_1 and vitamin K_2 reduced bone loss, but vitamin K_2 was significantly more effective, reducing risk of vertebral fracture by 60%, hip fracture by 77%, and all nonvertebral fractures by 81%.[168]

Numerous other recent studies have also shown that supplementation with vitamin K, particularly vitamin K_2, improves bone mineral density, helps protect against osteoporosis, and helps women with osteoporosis rebuild healthy bone.[169]

Vitamin K_2 Partners with Vitamin D_3

Another reason to take vitamin K_2 is that K_2 partners with vitamin D. Vitamin D increases the production of osteocalcin and matrix-Gla protein, both of which require vitamin K_2 to become activated. Vitamin D thus increases both the demand for vitamin K_2 and the potential for benefit from K_2-dependent proteins.

Not surprisingly, the combination of vitamin K_2 and vitamin D_3 has been shown to be more effective in preventing bone loss than either nutrient alone. In a study of 173 osteoporotic/osteopenic women, those given both K_2 and D_3 experienced an average 4.92% increase in bone mineral density (BMD), while K_2 alone resulted in an average BMD increase of just 0.13%.[170]

The combined use of K_2 and D_3 has also been found to be more effective than either nutrient alone in improving bone mineral density (BMD) in postmenopausal women. In a 2-year study, 92 postmenopausal women were assigned to one of four groups: K_2 (45 milligrams per day of the menaquinone-4 form), D_3 (3,000 IU per day), a combination of these dosages of K_2 and D_3, or calcium lactate (2 grams per day). In the women receiving only calcium lumbar BMD decreased. Those given either D_3 or K_2 experienced a slight increase in BMD, but those taking both K_2 and D_3 fared much better, increasing BMD in the lumbar spine (the part of the spine between the diaphragm and the pelvis) by 1.35%.[171]

How Much Do I Need?

You may be wondering, "Can I get enough vitamin K_2 to produce healthy bones from the K_1 and K_2 in my diet?" Probably not, even if you eat several cups of leafy greens every day.

Here's why: because ensuring that your blood will clot is more important for your immediate survival needs than putting calcium into your bones (or keeping it out of your arteries), all the vitamin K_1 in the foods you consume will first be used to activate the proteins necessary for blood clotting.[172] Only after this need has been met will any K_1 that is left over be available for conversion to K_2. In a best case scenario, only about 6% of the K_1 in the leafy greens you eat will ultimately get converted to K_2, and this means not enough K_2 for healthy bones (for an estimate of just how little K_2 this is, see the table on the next page).

In addition, whether you can convert K_1 to K_2 also depends upon whether you have healthy intestines, well supplied with the probiotic bacteria that do this job. If you have any gastrointestinal problems, your ability to produce K_2

FOOD SOURCES OF VITAMIN K₁[173]

Food	Serving	Micrograms of Vitamin K₁	Amount in micrograms potentially converted to K₂ (MK-4 form)
Kale, raw	1 cup, chopped	547 mcg	32 mcg
Swiss chard, raw	1 cup	299 mcg	18 mcg
Parsley, raw	1/4 cup	246 mcg	15 mcg
Broccoli, cooked	1 cup, chopped	220 mcg	13 mcg
Spinach, raw	1 cup	145 mcg	9 mcg
Watercress	1 cup, chopped	85 mcg	5 mcg
Green leaf lettuce, raw	1 cup, shredded	63 mcg	4 mcg
Soybean oil	1 tablespoon	25 mcg	2 mcg
Canola oil	1 tablespoon	17 mcg	1 mcg
Olive oil	1 tablespoon	8 mcg	0.5 mcg
Mayonnaise	1 tablespoon	4 mcg	0.2 mcg

may be greatly reduced, even if you are eating lots of foods rich in K_1.

So, do you eat lots of leafy greens every day? If you do, and your digestive system is well supplied with probiotic bacteria, you may be providing your bones with a tiny amount of K_2. But here's where it gets a bit more complicated because vitamin K_2 comes in two different flavors, menaquinone-4 (MK-4), and menaquinone-7 (MK-7). Humans typically convert K_1 into the MK-4 form of K_2, producing, at best, microgram amounts. But the research shows that, for healthy bones, we need at least 45 *milligrams* of MK-4, or much less (1,000 times less!), 45 *micrograms*, of MK-7.[174]

Both forms of K_2, MK-4 and MK-7, are found in certain foods, but in amounts too small for us to rely on them to protect our bones. MK-4 is found in the fat in some animal products (dairy products like cheese and egg yolk), while menaquinone-7 (MK-7) is present in fermented foods, such as sauerkraut and a fermented soybean product available in Japan called "natto." Unfortunately, natto is the only food that contains enough MK-7 to meet our bones' needs (approximately 870 micrograms per 3 ounces[175]). I say "unfortunately" because not only is natto hard to find in the US, it is an acquired taste, even in Japan, due to its slimy texture and, for many people, pungent, unpalatable flavor.

Thus, to ensure the health of your bones, it is simplest and safest to take a supplement that supplies K_2, either in the form of MK-4, for which you will need to take 45 milligrams (15 mg, three times per day), or in the form of MK-7, for which *at least* 45 micrograms is recommended. Higher doses, ranging from 180 micrograms to 865 micrograms, have been shown in several recent studies, to be more effective. A randomized, double-blind study conducted on 35 lung and 59 heart transplant recipients during the first year after organ transplantation (transplant recipients are at greatly increased risk for osteoporosis) found a 180 microgram per day dose of MK-7 helpful in protecting lumbar spine bone mineral density (BMD).[176] And, a recent review of research on food factors shown to prevent osteoporosis found that people consuming 1.5 ounces of "reinforced natto" that provided 865 micrograms of MK-7 per day had much higher levels of activated osteocalcin than people consuming regular natto, which contains about 435 micrograms of MK-7 in 1.5 ounces.[177]

In January 2001, the US Food and Nutrition Board of the Institute of Medicine established an adequate intake (AI) level for vitamin K_1 of 90 micrograms per day for women and 120 micrograms per day for men.[178] The published research has shown this is way too little to promote optimal bone health.

What to Look For in a Supplement

The research shows that for healthy bones, we need 45 milligrams of MK-4 but less than 1 milligram of MK-7 daily. Why? What's the difference between these two forms of vitamin K_2?

Commercially available MK-4 is produced synthetically. This is the form that has been most widely used in the research. However, although it is well absorbed and gets into the bloodstream quickly, MK-4 has a half-life of only 1–2 hours. For this reason, high pharmacological doses (typically 45 milligrams per day, divided into 3 daily doses of 15 milligrams each) are necessary. This not only makes it inconvenient to take, but such high doses necessitate medical supervision in patients on blood-thinning medications (e.g., warfarin).

MK-7, a natural compound derived from natto, is also very well absorbed, and as little as 45 micrograms per day has been found to activate sufficient osteocalcin for bone health, although recent studies indicate doses ranging from 180 micrograms to 865 micrograms per day may be more effective. Less MK-7 is needed because this form of the vitamin hangs around a lot longer than MK-4; MK-7 has a serum half-life of 3 days, which enables the body to build up a buffer that can supply vitamin K2 to all tissues 24 hours a day. MK-4 has a serum half-life of 6-8 hours. Even the highest dose of MK-7 shown effective in the research (865 micrograms/day) is much smaller than the dose required for MK-4 (45 mg, which, in the studies, is taken as three 15 mg doses throughout the day). The smaller dose not only makes MK-7 easier to take, but renders it highly unlikely to interact negatively with blood-thinning medications.[179]

Safety Issues

None. No adverse effects have been reported for higher levels of vitamin K intake from food and/ or supplements, and there are no documented toxicity symptoms for vitamin K. In animal studies, vitamin K in amounts as high as 25 micrograms per kilogram of body weight per day (the equivalent of 1,750 micrograms of vitamin K for an adult human weighing 154 pounds) has produced no noticeable toxicity. Thus, when the Institute of Medicine at the National Academy of Sciences published its health recommendations for this nutrient in 2001, the experts chose not to set a Tolerable Upper Limit (UL) for vitamin K.[180]

B VITAMINS (B$_6$, B$_{12}$, FOLATE, AND RIBOFLAVIN)

What They Do

As mentioned earlier in the section **"Bs" for Better Bones**,* the B vitamins are needed to prevent levels of homocysteine, a nasty middleman compound in a very important cellular process called methylation, from accumulating.

Collagen is the main protein component in our bones. Collagen proteins link together, forming the organic part of the bone matrix. Homocysteine interferes with collagen cross-linking, causing a defective bone matrix and increased bone fragility.[181] In cell studies, homocysteine has been shown to trigger the self-destruct sequence (called *apoptosis*) in the cells that build bone (osteoblasts), and to increase the formation and activity of the cells that break down bone (osteoclasts).[182]

In addition to these directly harmful effects on bone, elevated homocysteine also promotes chronic inflammation, which triggers osteoclast

---

* See page 68.

production and activity, a significant contributing factor to bone loss in older individuals, particularly postmenopausal women. (Osteoclasts are the target of the bisphosphonate patent medicines, which were designed to help maintain bone mass by poisoning osteoclasts.)

Also as mentioned earlier,* estrogen helps lessen inflammation, which is one of the key reasons its decline during menopause results in increased bone loss.[183] When adequate supplies of the B vitamins are present, homocysteine is quickly metabolized into a harmless compound.

What to Look For in a Supplement

The following amounts should be present in a day's recommended dose of your multiple vitamin. Note that a daily dose of some multiple vitamins may be 2, 3, or even as many as 6 capsules. The *total* amount of the B vitamins provided by the daily dose should be at least:

- B_6: 50 milligrams
- B_{12}: 500 micrograms

---

* In the "What It Does" section for vitamin K, page 141.

- Folate: 1,000 micrograms
- Riboflavin: 50 milligrams

Safety Issues

B_6: Nervous system imbalances have been shown to result from very high levels of vitamin B_6 intake—more than 2 grams (2,000 milligrams) per day. The tolerable Upper Intake Level (UL) set for vitamin B_6 for adults 19 years and older by the National Academy of Sciences is 100 milligrams per day.

Folate: At doses greater than 1,000–2,000 micrograms, "inactive synthetic folate" (the fully oxidized, inactive "folic acid" form of folate obtained from supplements and/or fortified foods) can trigger nervous system-related symptoms, including insomnia, malaise, irritability, and intestinal dysfunction. The UL set for folic acid by the Institute of Medicine at the National Academy of Sciences is 1,000 micrograms for adults 19 years and older. As this is being written, most suppliers of multivitamins are switching from the inactive folic acid to the active methylfolate and folinic acid (or calcium folinate) forms. If at all possible, use one of these.

B_{12}: No toxicity symptoms have been reported for B_{12}, even in long-term studies in which subjects took 1,000 micrograms daily for 5 years, so the National Academy of Sciences has set no UL for B_{12}.

Riboflavin: No toxic side effects have been documented for riboflavin, so the National Academy of Sciences has not set a UL for riboflavin.

VITAMIN C

What It Does

As noted earlier in the section "'C' Your Way to Stronger Bones,"* vitamin C is essential for the development and maintenance of strong bones because 90% of the protein in the bone matrix is collagen, and vitamin C is an essential cofactor required for collagen formation. Vitamin C stimulates the production of osteoblasts (the cells that build bone), and is also one of the

---

* See page 76.

body's key antioxidants and thus helps lessen inflammation, which, if uncontrolled, results in increased production and activation of osteo-clasts, the cells that break down bone.[184]

What to Look For in a Supplement

Vitamin C, ascorbic acid, is very inexpensive and readily available. Your main concern is dosage. In postmenopausal women, greater bone mineral density has been reported when vitamin C intake from supplements increased from 0 to 500 to 1,000 milligrams per day. Higher intake of vitamin C has also been associated with significantly higher BMD (less bone loss) in older men who had never smoked.[185]

Look for a supplement that will allow you to take at least 1,000 milligrams per day, preferably 2,000 milligrams per day, without having to swallow several large hard pills. Capsules containing vitamin C powder, a jar of vitamin C powder, or a product like Emergen-C® (which provides vitamin C in 1,000-milligram packets, comes in a variety of flavors, and makes a pleasant tasting fizzy drink, may be better absorbed and easier to swallow than large, hard tablets. You can even use your Emergen-C® drink as the liquid with which to swallow your other supplements. Vitamin C powder will add a lemony tang to a glass of water, fruit juice, or cup of tea.

A very few individuals experience loose stools, gas, or even diarrhea, when taking a single 1,000 milligram dose of vitamin C. If you are one of them, you have two options: you can try taking a "buffered" version of vitamin C or you can take your vitamin C in divided doses. Buffered vitamin C powder usually combines ascorbic acid with minerals like calcium, magnesium, or potassium. When buffered vitamin C powder is mixed with water, the result is a reduced-acid solution that effervesces for a short while—a plus if you enjoy fizzy drinks—and won't irritate a sensitive stomach or intestinal lining.

Another option, Ester-C™, is a complex of ascorbic acid combined with several of its naturally occurring metabolites, including dehydroascorbate, threonate, and aldonic acids. Ester-C™ is significantly more expensive than plain old ascorbic acid, but it may be worth the additional cost. A test tube study found that cells treated with this vitamin C complex produced more collagen and mineralized tissue than cells treated with ascorbic acid alone, suggesting that Ester-C™ may be more effective in helping to promote bone regeneration than ascorbic acid.[186]

Safety Issues

In 2000, the National Academy of Sciences set a Tolerable Upper Intake Level (UL) for vitamin C at 2,000 milligrams (2 grams) for adults 19 years or older. This UL is probably too low.

Very few research studies document vitamin C toxicity at any level of supplementation, and no toxicity effects have ever been documented in relation to vitamin C from food in the diet. As mentioned, some persons react to high supplemental doses, typically involving 5 or more grams of vitamin C, by developing loose stools or diarrhea. This type of diarrhea is called "osmotic diarrhea" because it results from an excess of fluid concentrating in the intestine as the body attempts to dilute the amount of vitamin C present. The magnesium in Milk of Magnesia has the same effect.

Vitamin C can increase a person's absorption of iron from plant foods, such as spinach. Usually, this is beneficial, given that approximately 1 in 24 Americans or 11.2 million people in the USA, including 20% of premenopausal women and 2% of adult men, are iron-deficient.[187] However, those at risk of having excess free iron in their cells (e.g., men who eat a lot of red meat) may want to have their iron levels checked and donate blood or consider avoiding high supplemental doses of vitamin C.

Bone-Building Minerals

CALCIUM

What It Does

One of the most abundant minerals in the human body, calcium accounts for approximately 1.5% of total body weight, and approximately 99% of that calcium is stored in our bones and teeth.[188] The remaining 1%, however, is needed for numerous actions required for our physical bodies to continue to function. For example, calcium is necessary for blood clotting, neurotransmitter release, nerve conduction, and muscle contraction (including the contraction of the heart muscle—our heartbeat). Calcium regulates enzyme activity and cell membrane function, which determines what gets into and out of our cells.

Because these physiological activities are essential to life, our body has developed complex regulatory systems that tightly control the amount of calcium in the blood to ensure enough calcium is always available for them. When we don't consume enough calcium to maintain these essential blood levels, our body will draw on calcium stashed in our bones to maintain normal blood concentrations. Just like with any banking system, too many withdrawals without enough deposits leads to bankruptcy, which in the case of our bones, after many years, equals osteoporosis and bone fractures.

Calcium is best known for its role as the primary component that gives our bones strength and density. To mineralize bone, calcium joins with phosphorus, forming calcium phosphate, which then serves as the major component of the mineral complex—called *hydroxyapatite*—that provides structure and strength in bones.

Numerous studies have shown that calcium supplementation improves bone density in perimenopausal women and slows the rate of bone loss in postmenopausal women by 30 to 50%, significantly reducing the risk of hip fracture.[189] However, the most recent Cochrane Review (the gold standard in medical research) found that calcium supplementation *alone* has only a small positive effect on bone density.[190] This is the key point we are trying to make in this book! Healthy bones are the result not of just one, two, or even several compounds, but of more than a dozen nutrients derived from a healthy diet, supplements when optimal amounts of specific nutrients are difficult to get from the diet, and a healthy lifestyle that includes regular exercise.

What to Look For in a Supplement

Despite calcium's widespread availability in a variety of foods, most Americans are not getting enough to support healthy bones for life.* Thus, to ensure bone health, it's best to supplement. But how do you choose which of the many different available forms of supplemental calcium will best serve you? Here's what you need to know to decide.

Naturally-derived calcium: may appear on labels as bone meal, oyster shell, limestone, or dolomite (clay). Since naturally derived calcium supplements have been found to contain concentrations of lead far exceeding the most recent criteria established to limit lead exposure (>1.5 μg/g), these forms are best avoided.[191]

Calcium carbonate: the most commonly used form in calcium supplements, and that used in OTC antacids (e.g., Tums®, Rolaids®, Maalox®) is less expensive, but not nearly as well absorbed as the forms of calcium discussed below, chelated calcium or hydroxyapaptite.

If you choose calcium carbonate, it is very important that it be taken with meals when you will be secreting hydrochloric acid. Why? Calcium

---

* For a discussion of food sources of calcium, see "Are You Sure You're Getting Enough Calcium?," page 50.

is absorbed in the small intestine where normally, the pH balance is not acidic; therefore, stomach acid is needed not to absorb calcium, but to dissolve the delivery form—which in the case of calcium carbonate is essentially a piece of chalk.

Of concern is the fact that people with low stomach acid absorb only about 4% of an oral dose of calcium carbonate, and studies have found that about 40% of postmenopausal women are deficient in stomach acid. Obviously, if you do not have adequate stomach acid, antacids will not provide an effective means of delivering supplemental calcium to your bones![192]

What Might Cause You to Have Too Little Stomach Acid?

Two very common possibilities are infection with *Helicobacter pylori*, the pathogenic bacterium that promotes ulcers, and self- or doctor-prescribed medication with H2-blockers [e.g., cimetidine (Tagamet®), ranitidine (Zantac®), famotidine (Pepcid®), and nizatidine (Axid®)] or proton-pump inhibitors for heartburn or gastro-esophaegal reflux (GERD) [e.g., esomeprazole

(Nexium®), omeprazole (Prilosec®), lansopra-zole (Prevacid®), pantoprazole (Protonix®), rabe-prazole (Aciphex®)].

About 25% of the population in the western world, including North America, is infected with *H.pylori*. In developing nations, *H.pylori* infection is much more common, affecting upwards of 80% of the populations.[193] If you are taking any of the acid-blocking patent medicines listed, your likelihood of not having enough stomach acid to absorb the calcium from calcium carbonate is quite high.

Another common cause of low stomach acid is simply getting older. By the time both men and women reach age 60, half of us don't make enough acid in our stomachs to optimally digest all our food—and that includes dissolving the carbonate form of calcium. Other less common causes of low stomach acid include food allergy (especially dairy), overindulgence in alcohol, and the aftereffects of some viral illnesses.*

---

* For a complete discussion of low stomach acid, see *Your Stomach* by Dr. Wright, Praktikos Books: Mt. Jackson, VA, 2009.

Chelated calcium: will appear on the label as calcium citrate, calcium malate, calcium gluconate, calcium aspartate, etc. In these chelated forms, calcium is bound to either an organic acid (e.g., citrate, malate, gluconate) or amino acid (aspartate).

The resulting compounds are optimal calcium-delivery agents. They are 22% to 27% better absorbed than calcium carbonate; degrade almost completely even when stomach acid is relatively low (so they can be taken without food and are the supplement of choice for individuals with low stomach acid and those using stomach acid-blocking patent medicines), and do not contain lead or other toxic metals. Chelated forms have been shown to increase absorption of not only calcium, but other bone-building minerals such as magnesium.[194]

Hydroxyapatite: sometimes appears as MCHC (microcrystalline hydroxyapatite). The most expensive form of calcium, hydroxyapatite is a complex crystalline compound in which calcium is linked with phosphorus in a preformed building block of the bone mineral matrix.

FOODS RICH IN CALCIUM[195]

Food	Serving Size	Calcium (in milligrams)
Yogurt, low-fat	1 cup	447 mg
Sardines	1 each	351 mg
Sesame seeds	1/4 cup	351 mg
Goat's milk	1 cup	325 mg
Cow's milk	1 cup	297 mg
Spinach	1 cup	245 mg
Cabbage, shredded, cooked	1/2 cup	239 mg
Mozarella cheese, part-skim	1 oz	183 mg
Cottage cheese, 2%	1 cup	155 mg
Blackstrap molasses	2 teaspoons	118 mg
Mustard greens, steamed	1 cup	104 mg
Tofu	4 oz	100 mg
Broccoli	1 cup	75 mg
Cinnamon, dried, ground	2 teaspoons	56 mg
Thyme, dried, ground	2 teaspoons	54 mg
Oranges	1	52 mg
Oregano, dried, ground	2 teaspoons	47 mg
Romaine lettuce	2 cups	40 mg

MCHC contains hydroxyapatite plus bone-derived growth factors and all the trace minerals that comprise healthy bone. Although research on hydroxyapatite as a source of calcium is limited, two studies have shown it to be more effective in the prevention of osteoporosis caused by taking corticosteroid patent medicines.[196] And a recent meta-analysis of 12 well controlled trials comparing hydroxyapatite to calcium carbonate to prevent bone loss found hydroxyapatite increased bone mineral density 102% more than calcium carbonate![197]

Safety Issues

Consuming more than 3,000 milligrams of calcium per day could result in elevated blood levels of calcium, a condition called *hypercalcemia*. If blood levels of phosphorus are low when calcium levels are high, or if insufficient vitamin K_2 is available,* hypercalcemia can lead to calcification of soft tissues, including the arteries, heart, breasts, and kidneys. The

---

* See "Vitamin K," page 141.

Tolerable Upper Intake Level (UL) set for calcium, by the National Academy of Sciences in 1997, is 2,500 milligrams per day.

BORON

What It Does

Boron has been shown in numerous studies to have beneficial effects on bone architecture and strength.[198] Boron is a "trace mineral" meaning our bodies need just a trace to function properly; in boron's case, this is just 3–5 milligrams a day. But our bones really need that little bit because boron is required for the conversion of estrogen into its most active form, 17-beta-estradiol, and this is the form in which estrogen increases our bones' absorption of magnesium. Another key mineral in our bones, magnesium,* along with calcium and phosphorus, forms the crystal lattice structure of our bones.

Boron is also necessary for the reaction that occurs in the kidneys in which vitamin D is converted into its most active form [$1,25(OH)_2D_3$].

---

* See "Magnesium," page 173.

Estrogen increases the activity of our bone-building cells, the osteoblasts, and vitamin D is necessary for calcium absorption.[199]

When the US Department of Agriculture conducted an experiment in which postmenopausal women took 3 mg of boron a day, boron reduced the women's excretion of calcium by 44%, and also resulted in the activation of the bone-building forms of estrogen and vitamin D.[200]

What to Look For in a Supplement

Boron is one of the micronutrients your bones need for which a supplement is your best option. Although present in some foods, including raisins, hazelnuts, almonds, dried apricots, avocado, dates, peanuts, prunes, and walnuts, the amount of boron, even in these foods in which this trace mineral is most concentrated, is really small. Raisins are the richest food source of boron, and you'd have to eat 3 ounces of raisins (185 calories worth) to gain 4.5 mg of boron. Three ounces (6 tablespoons, which deliver 570 calories and 48 grams of fat) of peanut butter will give you less than 2 milligrams of boron.

Eat this amount of peanut butter every day and you can forget zipping up your jeans. Supplementation is obviously a more practical and less "weighty" means of receiving the daily 3–5 mg of boron you need for optimal bone health.

Safety Issues

None. Elemental boron and borates are nontoxic to humans, animals, or fish. The *LD50* (which is the dose of a compound high enough to kill 50% of animals tested) is about 6 grams per kilogram of body weight. Substances whose LD50 is greater than 2 grams are considered nontoxic. In humans, intake of 4 grams per day was reported to cause no incidents, and medical dosages of 20 grams of boric acid have caused no problems. The Tolerable Upper Intake Level (UL), the maximum dose at which no harmful effects would be expected, is 20 mg per day for adults and pregnant or breastfeeding women over 19 years of age.[201]

MAGNESIUM

What It Does

Magnesium is classified as a "macro-mineral" because it plays so many roles in our bodies that we need several hundred milligrams every day. Magnesium activates more than 300 enzymes, is involved in the production of ATP (the energy currency of the body), and serves as a key compound in the crystal latticework matrix that gives structure to our bones. One of the enzymes activated by magnesium is involved in the conversion of vitamin D into its most active form—the form in which vitamin D greatly increases our ability to absorb calcium.

About two-thirds of the magnesium in our bodies goes into our bones, which serve as the body's bank account for magnesium, just as they do for calcium. When we are under stress—a not uncommon occurrence in our modern, excessively busy lives—our bodies use up magnesium at a very rapid clip.[202] Our hectic, stressful lives may translate into a need for more magnesium than the Adequate Intake (AI) recommended in 1997 by the Institute of

Medicine at the National Academy of Sciences, which was a daily 360 milligrams for women or 400 milligrams for men. Among women in the US, the average dietary intake of magnesium is only 68% of this possibly insufficient AI, which means that a very large proportion of American women are deficient in magnesium.[203]

When our magnesium levels drop too low, so do our blood levels of the most active form of vitamin D [$1,25(OH)_2D_3$], which plays a key role in our ability to absorb calcium.[204] In addition, an increase occurs in a compound called "skeletal substance P," which promotes inflammation and bone breakdown.[205]

Magnesium is also necessary for regulating the secretion of parathyroid hormone and calcitonin—the two hormones responsible for maintaining the proper concentration of calcium within our bloodstream. When calcium levels are too low, parathyroid hormone stimulates osteoclasts to break down bone, thus increasing blood calcium levels. When calcium levels are too high, calcitonin suppresses the activity of osteoclasts, the cells that break down bone.

FOODS RICH IN MAGNESIUM[206]

Food	Serving Size	Magnesium (in milligrams)
Pumpkin seeds	1/4 cup	185 mg
Spinach, steamed	1 cup	157 mg
Soybeans	1 cup	148 mg
Swiss chard, steamed	1 cup	150 mg
Halibut	4 oz	121 mg
Salmon, Chinook	4 oz.	138 mg
Navy beans	1 cup	107 mg
Almonds	1/4 cup	99 mg
Pinto beans	1 cup	94 mg
Cashews	1/4 cup	89 mg
Scallops	4 oz	77 mg
Tuna, yellowfin	4 oz	73 mg
Flaxseeds	2 tablespoons	70 mg
Summer squash	1 cup	43 mg
Beets, cooked	1 cup	39 mg
Broccoli, steamed	1 cup	39 mg
Brussels sprouts	1 cup	31 mg
Green beans	1 cup	31 mg
Banana	1 medium	29 mg
Whole wheat bread	1 slice	28 mg
Kiwi fruit	1	22 mg
Tomato, ripe	1 cup	20 mg

Thus, not having enough magnesium on board translates into impaired ability to absorb calcium and regulate its levels in the bloodstream, which leads to an increase in bone loss, plus a reduction in our body's ability to form new bone. Not surprisingly, women with osteoporosis have been shown to have a lower level of magnesium in their bones and to have other indications of magnesium deficiency compared to people without osteoporosis.[207]

A final consideration—supplementing with vitamin D may increase your magnesium needs. Calcium and magnesium counterbalance one another in numerous cellular activities. If you are taking vitamin D, you will be absorbing more calcium, so you will also need more magnesium to maintain the balance between these minerals, both of which are vitally important for your overall health as well as that of your bones.

Symptoms of magnesium insufficiency include migraines and tension headaches, muscle weakness, leg cramps, restless legs, elevated blood pressure, transient ischemic attacks, and arrhythmia. If you are going to regularly be taking more than 2,000 IU/day of vitamin D, an amount that the latest research shows most of us need to maintain healthy blood levels of this vitamin, then you should consider supplementing with magnesium.

What to Look For in a Supplement

For the same reasons that choosing a supplement providing calcium in a chelated form is recommended above,* a chelated form of magnesium will serve you best. Look for products containing magnesium citrate, magnesium malate, or magnesium aspartate. Take 250 milligrams, twice daily.

In the unlikely event that you develop loose stools from supplementing with magnesium, try taking 25 milligrams of *pyridoxal-5-phosphate* (P5P) along with the magnesium. P5P is the activated form of vitamin B_6 and is responsible for ferrying magnesium inside your cells. In some people, the enzyme that converts B_6 into P5P is underactive, either because of their genetic inheritance or because they are lacking in riboflavin, which is also involved in this conversion. In either case, this can result in

---

* See "Chelated calcium," page 167.

difficulty absorbing magnesium, which can be remedied by taking P5P.[208]

Safety Issues

Intake of high levels of supplemental magnesium may cause diarrhea. This symptom has been noted in research studies in which doses of magnesium ranged from 1–5 grams (1,000–5,000 milligrams) but, as noted above, diarrhea can occur at lower supplemental doses.

If this happens, it may be due to impaired conversion of vitamin B_6 to its active form, P5P, which is responsible for bringing magnesium inside our cells. Supplying P5P by taking a P5P supplement providing 25 milligrams may greatly improve the body's ability to absorb magnesium. The upper tolerable limit set for supplemental magnesium by the National Academy of Sciences in 1997 is 350 milligrams per day for individuals 9 years or older.

STRONTIUM

What It Does

In just the last five years, more than 400 articles have been published in the peer-reviewed medical literature on the bone-building effects of strontium. One of the most abundant minerals on earth, strontium is present in the soil, air, water, fish, and most plant foods, especially cabbage, beets, and Brazil nuts. Worldwide, humans' estimated daily intake of strontium is 1–5 milligrams per day.

Chemically similar to calcium, strontium is absorbed in comparable amounts. Once in bone, strontium beneficially affects both aspects of the bone remodeling process: it not only slows down the development of osteoclasts, thus lessening bone removal activity, but also enhances the development of osteoblasts, thus increasing bone-forming activity.

Since pure strontium is chemically unstable, it is found in Nature in the form of salts, such as strontium citrate, strontium chloride, strontium carbonate, strontium gluconate, or strontium lactate. Strontium ranelate, a recently created, new-to-nature patentable form, has been the subject of a number of large, double-blind, placebo-controlled trials (further discussed below), which have confirmed strontium's effectiveness in halting and reversing osteoporosis. Strontium ranelate combines strontium with a synthetic compound called ranelic acid, which is supposed to be very poorly absorbed. This patentable form of strontium is currently being marketed in Europe (trade name Protelos®) for the prevention and treatment of osteoporosis.

Strontium's ability to prevent early postmenopausal bone loss was evaluated in a 24-month double-blind placebo-controlled study of 160 postmenopausal women. All the women were given calcium (500 milligrams per day). Those who also received strontium ranelate (1 gram per day) increased their lumbar BMD by an average of 5.53% compared to the women who were given a placebo. After two years, bone mineral density in the femoral neck (the neck-shaped area near the top of the femur) had increased 2.46% and BMD in the hip had increased 3.21%

in women given strontium ranelate compared to those given the placebo. Plus, strontium was as well tolerated as the placebo.[209]

Strontium was also shown to greatly benefit postmenopausal women who had already had a vertebral osteoporotic fracture. In a two-year, double-blind, placebo-controlled trial involving 353 Caucasian women, study participants were given either strontium ranelate (0.5, 1, or 2 grams per day) or a placebo. All the women also received a daily 500-milligram supplement of calcium along with an 800 IU vitamin D_3 supplement. At the end of the study, the yearly increase in lumbar BMD in the women given 2 grams of strontium ranelate was 7.3%. During the second year of treatment, the 2-gram dose was associated with a 44% reduction in the number of patients who experienced a new vertebral fracture. Treating postmenopausal women who already had osteoporosis with strontium ranelate (2 grams daily for two years) resulted in an increase in these women's lumbar BMD of about 3% each year.[210]

The largest, most significant study of strontium to date was a five-year study that began in 1996 and included two clinical trials evaluating strontium ranelate's effects on women with osteoporosis: (1) the spinal osteoporosis therapeutic intervention (SOTI) study, which had a study population of 1,649 patients (average age was 70 years) and looked at strontium's effects on the women's risk of vertebral fractures, and (2) the treatment of peripheral osteoporosis (TROPOS) trial, which included 5,091 patients (average age was 77 years) and looked at strontium's effects on nonspinal fractures. Both studies were multinational, randomized, double-blind, placebo-controlled trials that included two parallel groups: women with osteoporosis who were given strontium ranelate (2 grams per day) compared to a second comparable group of women with osteoporosis receiving a placebo.

After three years of follow-up, the SOTI study revealed that strontium caused a 41% reduction in the women's risk of experiencing a vertebral fracture compared to the placebo. Even in the first year, the women's risk of a new vertebral fracture was reduced 49% in the strontium group compared to the placebo. Lumbar BMD increased 11.4% in the strontium group, but decreased 1.3% in the placebo group. And strontium caused no adverse side effects.[211]

The TROPOS study, which looked at the effect of strontium on nonvertebral fractures, showed a reduction in risk of 16% in all vertebral fractures and a 19% reduction in risk of major nonvertebral osteoporotic fractures. In a subgroup of women at high risk of fracture—women 74 years of age or older who had a low femoral neck bone mineral density score—treatment with strontium was associated with a 36% reduction in risk of hip fracture.[212]

Strontium was also studied in 1,431 postmenopausal women with *osteopenia* (accelerated bone loss, an early warning signal for developing osteoporosis). In women with lumbar spine osteopenia, strontium ranelate decreased the risk of vertebral fracture by 41% (by 59% in women who had not yet experienced a fracture and by 38% in women who had already had a fracture). In women with osteopenia at both the lumbar spine and the neck of the femur, strontium reduced fracture risk by 52%.[213]

Most recently, a review found strontium was able to reduce vertebral fracture risk in patients with osteopenia, and to reduce vertebral, non-vertebral, and hip fractures in patients with osteoporosis aged 74 years and older.[214] A study involving 325 postmenopausal women with osteoporosis in mainland China, Hong Kong, and Malaysia, also confirmed strontium's benefits. After one year of taking either 2 grams of strontium or a placebo daily, bone mineral density in the lumbar spine, femoral neck, and hip in the women receiving strontium increased by 3–5% compared to those given the placebo.[215]

One more reason not to take a bisphosphonate: when a woman stops taking these patent medicines, bone remodeling remains suppressed for *at least* 6 months, which blunts bones' ability to benefit from strontium. A study published March 2010 in the *Journal of Bone Mineral Research* evaluated 120 women with osteoporosis in the United Kingdom, 60 of whom had taken bisphosphonates, and 60 of whom had not. All 120 women received strontium, calcium, and vitamin D. After one year, bone mineral density went up 5.6% at the spine, 3.4% at the hip, and 4.0% at the heel in the women who had *not* taken a bisphosphonate. In contrast, the women who had been on a bisphosphonate had only 2.1% increase at the spine and no increase in BMD at the hip or heel. Researchers do not know how long it will take for normal remodeling to begin again in the bones of the women who had used a bisphosphonate. [216]

What to Look For in a Supplement

How much strontium should you use? Based on the current research, it looks like somewhere between 340 and 680 milligrams of elemental strontium works best. The smaller quantities will help prevent bone loss from occurring while the larger doses can help treat osteoporosis.

In the US and Canada, natural strontium is available as an individual supplement, but you can also gain the benefits of strontium combined with other bone-building nutrients. Working with a company called Progressive Laboratories (800-527-9512, www.progressivelabs.com), Dr.

Wright has developed a formula called Osteo-Mins that combines strontium with other bone-building nutrients including calcium, magnesium, vitamin D, vitamin K, zinc, copper, boron, silicon, manganese, selenium, and molybdenum. Osteo-Mins is available through natural food stores, compounding pharmacies, and the Tahoma Clinic Dispensary.

Safety Issues

Strontium improves bone mineral density and strengthens bone in a normal, healthy way. This mineral is so safe that it is the key ingredient in toothpastes for sensitive teeth, such as Sensodyne®, which includes 10% total strontium chloride hexahydrate by weight. Strontium reduces tooth sensitivity by forming a barrier over microscopic tubules in tooth dentin in which nerve endings have become exposed by gum recession.[217]

However, since the quantities of strontium used in the studies are larger than those we might normally consume in our food each day, researchers wanted to check to be sure long-term use of strontium would not cause any alterations in the newly formed bone crystals or any other negative side effects. A number of studies have now addressed these concerns.

Strontium has been shown to improve vertebral bone density and strength in rats without altering bone stiffness, indicating that the improvement occurred without causing abnormal bone crystals. In monkeys, strontium both decreased bone resorption (loss) and increased bone synthesis. And in cell cultures, strontium not only increased the reproduction of bone-forming osteoblast cells, but also enhanced and increased the synthesis of collagen (the major protein in the bone matrix).[218] In patients with postmenopausal osteoporosis, data from two large, double-blind, placebo-controlled, multicenter trials of 5 years' duration, strontium greatly reduced risk of fractures without causing any adverse side effects other than a very occasional case of nausea or diarrhea. Data on patients who continued to receive strontium during an additional three-year extension of these trials indicates that strontium continued to provide protection against new vertebral and nonvertebral fractures for the eight years of therapy, improving bone mineral density at numerous sites, and increasing markers of bone formation while decreasing markers of bone resorption.[219]

The only precaution—a very important one—is to make sure you're taking more calcium than strontium: much older research in animals shows that if strontium intake exceeds calcium intake over a long period of time, the animals develop bone deformities. Also, you will surely be at less risk for potential side effects if you take a natural form of strontium rather than the patent medicine form, strontium ranelate.

Some Potential Problems with Strontium Ranelate

When researchers looked at the combined data from both the SOTI and TROPOS trials, they found strontium ranelate increased the yearly incidence of *venous thromboembolism* (blood clots) by 7%. They also found a few cases of *DRESS syndrome* (which stands for "drug reaction with eosinophilia and systemic symptoms syndrome" and is also known as "drug hyper-sensitivity syndrome"), but they discounted these as being too few to be a "real" problem. However, since death is a possible side effect of DRESS syndrome, for those affected, it is a very real, very serious side effect!

Symptoms of DRESS syndrome usually begin 1 to 8 weeks after exposure to the offending patent medicine. Classic symptoms include a widespread rash, fever, and involvement of one or more internal organs. Approximately 50% of patients will have hepatitis (liver inflammation), 30% will have eosinophilia (a high concentration of white cells in the blood—a marker of immune system activation), 10% will have nephritis (kidney inflammation), and 10% will have pneumonitis (lung inflammation).

DRESS syndrome is often severe and can result in death if not diagnosed early. In a manner reminiscent of the initial trickle of reports that gradually turned into a flood linking osteonecrosis of the jaw and increased femur fracture risk in women taking bisphosphonates, reports of strontium-ranelate-associated

DRESS syndrome and acute renal failure are starting to appear.[220]

Strontium is a trace element naturally present in the human body, so these potential side effects may be due to its combination with ranelic acid, even though it is supposed to be poorly absorbed. If you decide to take strontium ranelate, *immediately* stop taking this patent medicine if any suspicious major skin disorders occur within two months of starting treatment.

But why take this risk? Why use strontium ranelate, a new-to-nature patent medication rather than one of the naturally occurring, but unpatentable, salt forms of strontium? The natural salt forms of strontium consist of a single strontium atom plus one or two molecules of citrate, chloride, carbonate, gluconate, or lactate. Each molecule of strontium ranelate, however, contains two atoms of strontium plus one molecule of the new-to-nature compound, ranelic acid. Since strontium is the active agent in building bone, why expose yourself to *any* risk of adverse events or pay the increased expense of a patent medicine when natural forms of strontium are readily available?

If you decide to take strontium as an individual supplement, *just remember to take more calcium than strontium!*

Bioidentical Hormone Replacement Builds Bone

Both estrogen and progesterone play key roles in maintaining healthy bones. Estrogen suppresses the production of osteoclasts, the cells that break down bone; slows down the activity of already formed osteoclasts; curbs the production of inflammatory cytokines (small proteins secreted by immune system cells that promote inflammation-associated bone loss); and enhances the absorption of calcium and its retention in bone.[221]

As important as estrogen is to bone health, however, if you've read the earlier sections of this book, you know that simply lessening the rate at which bone is broken down or resorbed is only half of the equation. Maintaining healthy bones requires constantly rebuilding the bone that needs to be replaced—which is where progesterone comes in. Progesterone is responsible for boosting the production and activity of the cells that build new bone, the osteoblasts.

Progesterone levels begin to decline in women long before menopause—in some women, the drop in progesterone begins as early as their late 30s. By the time a woman reaches age 50, she may have lost as much as 75% of her youthful progesterone production.[222]

Even in young women, progesterone levels are normally low during the first half of the menstrual cycle. Progesterone production increases during the second half of the menstrual cycle (the luteal phase) after an egg is released from a follicle in the ovaries—an event called *ovulation*. After ovulation, the remains of the follicle join to form the *corpus luteum*, whose primary function is to secrete lots of progesterone, which prepares the uterine lining for the implantation of the egg, if fertilized. If no ovulation takes place—which happens more and more frequently as women enter perimenopause—no corpus luteum is produced, and only the small baseline amount of progesterone, which is made by the adrenal glands, is available.

Young women may also lack optimal levels of progesterone if they are using oral contraceptives (*aka* birth control pills).[223] Birth control pills come in two flavors—those containing only a patented version of estrogen, and those that combine the patented estrogen with another patent medicine, a new-to-Nature analog of progesterone called a progestin. (The dangers of progestins are outlined in the section following: *"Why Bioidentical Hormones Rather than Conventional, Patent Medicine Version of HRT?"*) Both types of birth control pill work by inhibiting follicular development and preventing ovulation. Thus, both types of birth control pills inhibit young women's natural production of progesterone.[224] In addition, cadmium, a toxic compound in cigarette smoke,* disrupts the ovaries' production of progesterone.[225] For these reasons, even young or perimenopausal women may be at risk of producing too little progesterone to promote healthy bone remodeling. In the Canadian Multicentre Osteoporosis Study, oral

---

* See earlier discussion on page 109.

contraceptive users had bone mineral density scores 2.3% to 3.7% lower than women who had never used oral contraceptives.[226]

Symptoms of premenopausal progesterone insufficiency may include: heavy periods, premenstrual syndrome (PMS), migraine and other headaches, fibrocystic breasts, breast tenderness, decreased libido, water retention/bloating, anxiety, and depression.

Since progesterone balances estrogen, opposing estrogen's stimulation of cell growth, insufficient progesterone translates into an increased risk of breast, uterine, and endometrial cancer. Because progesterone is necessary for the production and activation of osteoblasts, having too little promotes bone loss.

Ready to look into finding out whether your levels of estrogen and progesterone are adequate to protect your bones' health? It's easy to do so. Just ask your doctor to order a 24-hour urine collection hormone test for you.

Why Bother With a 24-Hour Urine Test When Saliva Tests Are Commonly Available by Mail Order and a Blood Draw Takes Only a Couple of Minutes?

Saliva test results are not reliable.[227] Blood tests are sometimes useful, but they only provide a snapshot of what's going on in your body at the moment the blood is drawn. 24-hour urine testing (yes, you collect your urine in a large bottle for a full 24 hours then transfer some samples to small vials for processing) is the preferred method of evaluating sex steroid hormone levels. It is the gold standard both because it is highly accurate and also because it provides way more information, including whether your hormones are being metabolized into helpful, safe compounds or into potentially cancer-causing ones. Neither saliva nor standard blood tests are able to measure many of these metabolites.[228]

One final caveat: be sure to work with a physician who will prescribe bioidentical hormone replacement for you if indicated.

Why Bioidentical Hormones Rather than Conventional, Patent Medicine Version of HRT?

Why use bioidentical hormones rather than the patent medicines, Premarin® (horse estrogens derived from the urine of pregnant mares) and Provera® (medroxyprogesterone, a patented, lab-created progestin—not progesterone!)?

Chances are you are already thinking the answer to this question is obvious! The bodies of postmenopausal women, including their bones, do better when given hormones identical to those their premenopausal bodies produced than when given those produced by female horses (conjugated equine estrogens, trade name Premarin®) or some unnatural aberration concocted in a chemistry lab (medroxyprogesterone, trade name Provera®).

Not only are bioidentical hormones more effective, but numerous studies have demonstrated that patented HRT is extremely dangerous. Perhaps the most widely publicized of these trials has been the Women's Health

Initiative (WHI). It was impossible to keep it quiet in 2002, when the WHI was halted early (after 5.2 years instead of its planned 8.5 years), because risks for both breast cancer and cardiovascular disease (heart attack, stroke, blood clots) went way up in the women who were receiving conventional HRT (Premarin® and Provera®).[229]

It's true that horse estrogens (conventional HRT) were found to offer a very small degree of protection against osteoporosis—5 to 7 fewer hip fractures per 10,000 women compared to a placebo.[230] But because patented HRT (Premarin®, Provera®, Prempro®—the last one being a pill that combines conjugated equine estrogens with medroxyprogesterone) have been definitively shown to increase your risk of cancer, heart disease, and stroke, conventional HRT is now primarily used to treat hot flashes and is prescribed at the lowest possible dose for the shortest amount of time possible.

One very positive result of the WHI's exposure of the risks of taking conventional HRT: its use—even short term for hot flashes—quickly plummeted by more than 50%. And as a result of this drop in the numbers of women taking HRT, the incidence of breast cancer fell 8.8% in women ranging in age from 40 to 79! [231]

Safety Issues

Too much estrogen—even bioidentical estrogen—can overstimulate cell growth in the lining of the uterus or breast. If you decide to investigate BHRT, read Dr. Wright's latest book on the subject, coauthored by Lane Lenard, PhD, *Stay Young & Sexy with Bio-Identical Hormone Replacement, the Science Explained*, and work with a physician well versed in this area.*

Prescriptions for bioidentical hormone replacement are not cookie cutter items. You will need to be tested to determine the estrogen dosage your body requires; a compounding pharmacy will then formulate a prescription specifically for you, and your doctor will monitor you using blood and urine tests at regular

---

* For help finding a physician in your area, see in Resources section: "Where Can I Find an 'Integrative' Doctor Who Will Help Me Build and Keep My Bones Strong, Naturally?"

intervals to ensure you are getting all the benefits without increasing cancer risk.

Your doctor will also help you determine how much bioidentical progesterone is optimal for you. Unlike estrogen, bioidentical progesterone is not a growth stimulator. During the short period in which your dose may need adjusting, too much might make you sleepy, but will not cause any unpleasant or dangerous side effects.

In contrast, the patent medicines containing progestins (Provera®, Prempro®), which are given with conjugated equine estrogens to supposedly help lessen the risk of unopposed estrogen, may not only cause breast tenderness, skin irritations, depression, breakthrough bleeding, swelling, and hirsutism (excessive hairiness in atypical areas, e.g., a mustache on a woman), but also contribute to conventional HRT's increased risk of asthma, stroke, heart disease, and breast, ovarian, and endometrial cancer.[232]

The claim to fame of the latest, fourth-generation progestins (e.g., drospirenone, dienogest), which are used in birth control pills, is that they have been designed to be closer in activity to the bioidentical progesterone (which raises the obvious question: why not just use bioidentical progesterone?), but their potential for causing coronary heart disease and breast cancer still remains an open question.[233]

No perimenopausal woman desiring to take progesterone to help prevent accelerated bone loss during the years immediately prior to menopause should have to subject herself to these risks when she can take bioidentical progesterone. Young women at increased risk for osteoporosis* may also wish to consider using alternative means of birth control, e.g., a cervical cap, diaphragm, or condom.

---

* See Chapter 1, page 3.

The Bone-Building Diet (I Can Eat My Way to Strong, Healthy Bones?)

You've probably heard the saying, "You are what you eat." It's true, particularly in relation to your bones. If you want strong, healthy bones for life, you've got to eat real food, mostly plants, preferably organic.

Conveniently, this healthy way of eating that creates and maintains strong bones for life is essentially the same diet that will lower your risk not only for osteoporosis, but for all chronic degenerative diseases, including cancer, diabetes, heart disease, and Alzheimer's.

Among all modern, technologically advanced Western societies, the lowest incidence of osteoporosis is found in the countries along the Mediterranean Sea, a fact attributed to the eating pattern in this area. If you want to put a label on it, you can call it the Bone-Building Mediterranean-Style Diet.[234]

It includes *lots of fresh vegetables* accompanied by:

- Beans
- Wild-caught fish
- Free-range eggs
- Low-fat dairy products, like yogurt, and a little cheese, often from goat's milk
- Small amounts of other animal protein, e.g., organically-raised free-range chicken, turkey, beef, pork
- Nuts and seeds
- Whole grains like brown rice, whole wheat pasta or bread, oats, quinoa
- Extra virgin olive oil as the primary source of added fat
- A wide variety of herbs and spices as seasonings
- Fruit, preferably fresh, for snacks and dessert
- If desired, one to two daily 4-ounce servings of red wine

In his book, *In Defense of Food*, Michael Pollan sums up how to follow the healthiest way of eating by saying: "Eat food. Not too much. Mostly plants."[235] To spotlight bone health, we just need to shift the emphasis to *what* rather than *how much*.

Happily, *"how much"* becomes a nonissue anyway since it's virtually impossible to consume too many calories when eating "real food, mostly plants, preferably organic"—unless you make like a squirrel preparing for hibernation and really pack away those nuts. A small handful of nuts, about an ounce a day, is the amount you should enjoy and not risk gaining too much weight.

You also need to limit your alcohol consumption.* One or even two 4-ounce glasses of red wine is a good idea. Red wine contains a bone-building, longevity-promoting phytonutrient called resveratrol, which has been shown to significantly promote osteoblast production and to prevent bone loss caused by estrogen deficiency.[236] However, if you drink more than 2 daily glasses of wine, as explained earlier, your bones will not be fine.†

---

* See page 115.

† See "More Than Two Drinks of Liquor Makes Bone Loss Much Quicker," page 115.

So, What Do the Three Catch-Phrases—Eat Real Food, Mostly Plants, Preferably Organic—Actually Mean?

Eat Real Food

Eat food as close to its natural state as possible. This means buy mostly food that is unprocessed, unpackaged, and unadulterated. This kind of food is found along the perimeter of the grocery store in the refrigerated sections.

Real food has to be refrigerated because, unlike the stuff in boxes in the aisles, it is not loaded with preservatives, fake flavoring, color additives, salt, sugars, etc., etc. Instead, real food is loaded with literally thousands of health-building nutrient compounds and enzymes that will quickly spoil on the shelf, but are needed to prevent our bodies, including our bones, from spoiling. These compounds are removed from the highly processed food-like items in the non-refrigerated aisles in our grocery stores to extend their "shelf life." If you prefer to extend your life, don't eat these.

Real food takes a little more time to prepare, but costs a lot less, even when organic. If you don't believe this, just compare the price of organic, thick-cut, rolled oats (1/4 cup will cook up into a large bowl of delicious hot oatmeal in about five minutes) to that of a packet of highly processed, sugar-and-chemical-laden instant oatmeal. Or compare the price of a large organic Russet potato to a bag of potato chips; if thinly sliced, tossed with a tablespoon of olive oil, spread on a cookie sheet, and baked, one potato will deliver the equivalent of a whole bag of potato chips, but for far fewer calories. Eating home-baked potato chips instead of that bag of overly processed, excessively greasy potato chips will shrink your waistline as well as your food bill. Plus, the olive oil you'll use to flavor them at home is good for your heart. The cheap, omega-6-rich (and therefore proinflammatory) oils used to process store-bought potato (and other) chips is not. Avoid proinflammatory, processed foods if you want to protect not only your heart and brain, but your bones.

If you have the space, consider planting a vegetable garden. Once you experience the taste of a just-picked snap pea, carrot, or vine-ripened tomato, or a tossed salad made from greens out of your own garden, you will be hooked. If you plant a vegetable garden, even if you pay more to buy vegetable starts rather than a packet of seeds, an investment of about $25 will provide an abundance of fresh produce from late spring through fall. You'll eat better, get a little exercise walking outside to the garden, and spend less.

A great resource for learning all you need to know to make choosing, storing, and cooking real food easy, practical, and delicious is the non-profit, totally free, no-advertisements website, The World's Healthiest Foods: www.whfoods.org.

Mostly Plants

Eat *at least* three cups of vegetables every day. Four to six cups would be good. Eight to ten cups would be better.

Eat lots of leafy greens. At the very least, one cup daily.* Going green every day helps keep

---

* See "Greens Give the Go-Ahead for Great Bones; Their Absence Slams the Brakes on Bone-Building," page 67.

osteoporosis away. An absence of greens in your daily diet slams the brakes on bone-building. For virtually no calories, green leafy vegetables deliver vast amounts of the minerals and vitamins your bones need, including calcium, magnesium, folate, vitamin C, and vitamin K_1. Fill up on leafy greens, and you will build up your bones, not your belly, hips, or thighs. And let's face it— you want not just great bones, but a great body, right? Greens will help you get both. Although green vegetables actually contain less calcium than many animal proteins, green vegetables contain very little if any phosphorus, which "offsets" the calcium. By contrast, animal proteins contain large quantities of phosphorus, which lead to excretion from our bodies of much of the calcium consumed in those animal proteins.

Not only do plant foods contain the nutrients necessary to build bone, but a diet rich in plant foods makes your body chemistry slightly alkaline, which is required for good bone health. As discussed earlier,* a diet high in animal protein

---

* See "Is Your Diet Leaching Calcium from Your Bones?," page 58.

promotes an acidic body chemistry. So does a diet high in refined sugars, including the high fructose corn syrup found in soft drinks and the vast majority of processed foods—yet another reason to avoid this junk. If protein or sugar dominates in your diet, your body will buffer the acidic chemistry produced by withdrawing alkaline minerals, i.e., calcium, from your bones.

Skimp on the refined sugars, but don't skimp on protein. Don't overdo it either.* This section also lists bone-friendly sources of protein. Bottom line, your best protein choices are low-fat dairy products; fish rich in omega-3 fatty acids but low in mercury, such as sardines and wild-caught salmon; calcium-enriched tofu; omega-3-rich free-range eggs; and beans.

Preferably Organic

Calorie-for-calorie, organically grown foods contain more bone-building minerals and phytonutrients than conventionally grown foods.

---

* See "How Much Protein Do YOU Need?" on page 59 to find out.

Nutrient levels in most conventionally grown fruits and vegetables have steadily declined, primarily as a result of what is called "the dilution effect." Conventionally grown crops grow bigger and faster as a result of the use of nitrogen fertilizer. Faster growing crops have less time to extract nutrients from the soil and move them up from the roots up the stalks and into the portions of the plant that are eaten.[237]

In addition, because they are protected by pesticides and constant irrigation from the stress caused by insects, fungal invasions, and drought, conventionally grown crops spend little energy on generating phytochemicals, including the vitamins and hundreds of health-promoting phenolic compounds plants can produce. Why? Because plants create these in response to their needs for self-defense. Less need = less self-defense nutrients in your food.[238]

Research confirms this. A review, released March 2008 by The Organic Center, identified 97 peer-reviewed studies published since 1980 that compared nutrient levels in organic and conventionally grown foods.[239] These studies were then rigorously analyzed for scientifically valid "matched pairs" of organic/conventionally grown produce. Two hundred and thirty-six matched pairs were found and evaluated for nutrient content. (To qualify as a matched pair, plants had to be grown nearby one another, in similar soils and climate, to have similar plant genetics, irrigation systems, nitrogen levels, and harvest practices.)

Organically grown fruits, vegetables, and grains were found to contain higher levels of eight of the eleven nutrients assayed, including higher levels of polyphenols and antioxidants. Overall, organically grown foods were 25% more nutrient-rich than conventionally grown varieties.

Not only was this difference found to be sizable enough to conclude organically grown foods can be counted upon to provide more nutrients, but Neal Davies, a Washington State University professor and a coauthor of the report, noted that "the nutrients in organically grown foods are often in a more biologically active form," which translates to more beneficial activity from the nutrient. In other words, the same amount of nutrient delivers more bang for the buck if consumed in an organically grown food.

In September 2009, a rebuttal to this study appeared in the *American Journal of Clinical Nutrition*. This paper, another review, discounted the claim that organically grown foods are nutritionally superior to conventionally grown. However, it wasn't a very good review. The reviewers did not use matched pairs and did not include antioxidant capacity in the compounds evaluated, in part because they relied upon much older studies starting back in 1958. These older studies analyzed plant varieties that are no longer even being cultivated and did not contain data on phenolic antioxidant compounds because they were just starting to be discovered!

Furthermore, the authors of this review made no allowance for the fact that since the 1950s, breeders and growers of nonorganic plants have used practices that have consistently increased yield but have lead to the dilution (lessening) of nutrients in the crop, as noted above.[240]

Since February 2008, fifteen new studies have been published, most of which utilize the updated design and superior analytical methods used in the Organic Center March 2008 review. These newer studies generally confirm the findings of the 2008 Organic Center report, particularly in the case of nitrogen (which is higher in conventional crops, a disadvantage since it may be converted into cancer-causing nitrates in the intestines), and for vitamin C, total phenolics, and total antioxidant capacity, which are typically higher in organically grown foods.[241]

An earlier review of 41 studies comparing organic to conventionally grown foods, published in 2002, found organically grown foods contained 27% more vitamin C, 21.1% more iron, 29.3% more magnesium, and 13.6% more phosphorus.[242]

A number of other current papers published in the peer-reviewed medical literature confirm that organic foods contain significantly higher levels of nutrients (especially bone-building vitamin C, polyphenols, flavonoids, and minerals) and lower levels of pesticides.[243]

And you really want to minimize your exposure to pesticides because they promote inflammation in humans, which, among their numerous other nasty effects, can contribute to bone loss by triggering osteoclast production and activity, and by causing mutations in hematopoietic stem cells—cells in bone marrow that give rise to all the different types of blood cells.[244]

A study comparing organic to conventionally grown tomatoes found organic tomatoes contained 4.52% more vitamin K, 129.81% more calcium, and 65.43% more zinc than conventionally grown tomatoes.[245]

Another, looking at celery, showed organic celery contained 70.22% more vitamin K, 47.93% more zinc, and 118.18% more vitamin C than conventionally grown celery.[246]

Yet another, analyzing the content of minerals and phenolic compounds in eggplant, found organic cultivation had such a positive effect on the accumulation of beneficial mineral and phenolic compounds that organically and conventionally produced eggplants could easily be told apart by looking at their nutrient composition profiles![247]

The nutritional profiles of a woman's diet—if she eats the high fat, high sugar, highly processed Standard American Diet (for which the shorthand is, aptly, SAD) or if she chooses a whole foods, mostly plants, mostly organic Mediterranean-style diet—will have a huge impact on what she will look and feel like at age 85. Don't be SAD! You can have strong, healthy bones for life. Eat a bone-building diet and you will greatly increase your likelihood of standing tall and looking good when you turn 85.

Bone-Building Exercises

Use It or Lose It

Lack of weight-bearing and resistance exercise is a well-documented risk factor for osteoporosis.[248] Numerous studies show that not moving against gravity—whether a result of being an astronaut on a space mission, in bed recovering from a surgery or illness, or life as a couch potato—leads to massive loss of bone minerals, as much as 1% of bone mineral mass per week![249]

On the other hand, in response to high-intensity and resistance exercise training, a number of studies of postmenopausal women have shown increases in bone mineral density that moved these women back toward the norm seen in healthy younger women.[250]

Typical gain in BMD after a year of regular exercise is 1–3%. Doesn't sound like all that much until you realize that, without exercise, women start losing BMD after age 40 at a rate of 0.3–0.5% per year. The rate of BMD loss increases after age 50 to about 1–1.5% per year, and is frequently more than 2% per year during the first 6–10 years after menopause, after which it slows back down to 1–2% per year.[251]

If regular exercise can give you a gain in BMD of 1–3% per year instead of a loss of 1–2% a year, it's actually preventing a 1–2% loss plus adding another 1–3% in BMD—this translates into an actual gain in BMD from exercise of 2–5% per year.

However, in studies in which postmenopausal women stopped exercising, the gains they made in spinal bone mineral density were lost after a period of inactivity. The message is clear: continue to use it or lose it.[252]

Why Is Exercise Essential for Healthy Bones as We Age?

Although our bones reach their full length (and we our full height) between the ages of 15 and 19, bones retain the capacity to grow in width throughout the human lifespan. With age, our bones thin and become more porous, but physical activity continues to stimulate increases in bone width and our bones' ability to absorb minerals for our entire lives. These exercise-stimulated increases in bone width and strength help offset aging's negative effects on bone.[253] In addition, regular physical exercise strengthens muscles and improves balance, thus greatly reducing risk of falls that could cause a fracture.[254]

While it is true that a postmenopausal woman's skeleton does not build bone as easily in response to exercise as that of a young woman, this is due primarily to the decline in female hormones (estrogen and progesterone) that occurs with menopause, and to inadequate intake of calcium, vitamin D, and the other nutrients involved in healthy bone formation (including vitamin C, vitamin K, the B vitamins, boron, magnesium, strontium). Fortunately, with bioidentical hormone replacement, a healthy diet, and supplemental bone-building nutrients, these lacks can easily be corrected.

What Kinds of Exercise and How Much Is Needed to Turn On Bones' Mineral-Absorbing, Width-Building Actions?

Unless you just love to exercise—yes, these people do exist—you're going to want to know what kinds of movement signal your bones to buff up and how many moves you have to make, so you can choose an exercise program that will deliver the goods in the least amount of time. Exercise physiologists now know that to build bone exercises must:[255]

Be dynamic, not static—Bones are designed to provide resistance against the forces of muscle contraction and gravity when body parts are moving. Rhythmic movement, such as dancing, walking briskly or jogging, climbing stairs (or using a StairMaster® or elliptical machine), lifting weights in a series of "sets" (e.g., six bicep or hamstring curls, a few seconds rest, six more curls, etc.); even sets of floor exercises, like sit ups or leg lifts, cause intermittent muscle contractions that deliver brief stresses on bone and increase blood supply to muscles, increasing delivery of nutrients, hormones, and oxygen. Static exercises—holding a yoga posture, floating on your back in the pool—while delivering other benefits, do not build bone. Swimming, although dynamic, is virtually gravity-free, so won't help build bone either.

Exceed a "threshold intensity"—After menopause, the effectiveness of exercise in increasing bone mineralization requires that it be not only regular but of sufficient intensity. Your bones have to get the message that you're working out! A leisurely stroll or window-shopping at the mall won't send it. We're talking "brisk walk" here. Speaking of which, if you can talk nonstop—stop! Then rev it up and use your breath to ramp up oxygen and nutrient delivery to your muscles, so you can build bone. In relation to weight lifting, if you can perform more than 4 sets of 8 reps of a bicep curl without feeling like your bicep muscle is on fire, you need to increase the weight.

Exceed a "threshold strain frequency"—The rate at which you contract your muscles counts. Increased frequency of contractions increases the bone-building response. Using dancing as an example, you want an upbeat, high tempo cha cha—not a waltz. You want to play tennis, not golf—well, golfing is okay if you forget the cart and walk really fast to the next spot where your ball ended up. (And carry your own clubs, too.) Get dewy—or just sweat. You can take a shower later.

Be relatively "brief and intermittent"—A couple of shorter, but gung ho, exercise sessions each day are much better than spending hours at the gym a couple of days a week. In fact, dividing your exercise time in half and exercising twice a day (say a half-hour before leaving for work or at lunch, and then another half-hour 6–8 hours later in the evening)—remember, energetic dancing counts—produces a more "osteogenic" (bone-building) response than spending your entire lunch hour or half of Saturday sloughing away. In other words, you can have a life, and still get enough exercise to make a real difference.

Impose an unusual "loading pattern" on the bones—You have to do something that uses different movement patterns and thus stresses your bones in uncustomary ways from your normal activities. The take home message here is don't do the same exercise routine over and over until you can breeze through it on auto-pilot, thinking about something else. Vary the order of the exercises or the way in which you work a muscle group. For example, if you lift weights, work a different muscle group first, use the machines in a different order, use free weights instead of machines, or find a different exercise than the one you usually do to work that muscle group. If you do Pilates mat work, add hand weights or use a prop like the Magic Circle to vary the exercise. For example, while doing the "100," put your lower legs inside the Circle and press your shins out, which will engage your outer thigh muscles. Next day, put the Circle between your lower shins and press in, strengthening your inner thighs, while doing the "100." If you always do the legwork after the Series of Five abdominal exercises, work your legs first, then do three of the Series of Five, then some back work, and then finish the abdominal exercises. If you are taking classes at a gym, you'll notice the good instructors do this anyway just to keep it interesting.

Be supported by adequate supplies of calcium and vitamin D₃—A key reason for exercise's bone-building effects is that exercise improves the body's ability to utilize vitamin D and calcium to build bone. If these nutrients aren't available then it's as if your bones got a call to go to a party, went to the closet, and *really* had nothing to wear. To build and maintain healthy bones, postmenopausal women need both calcium and exercise.

Studies have shown that neither calcium supplementation without exercise nor exercise without sufficient calcium intake can increase bone mineral density. Combine the two, however, and women's spinal BMD goes up.[256] It will go up a lot more if your bones are also receiving a good supply of all the other bone-building nutrients discussed earlier.

CHAPTER 8

If I Follow These Recommendations, What Can I Expect? How Soon Will I See Results?

BIOCHEMICAL TESTS OF BONE RESORPTION (BONE loss) should be run every three months until a normal reading is obtained. (Remember, after age 40, it's normal for both men and women to lose a tiny amount of bone each year, but the loss should be so small that it does not compromise bone strength.)

Initially, you should expect your rate of bone resorption to, at the very least, greatly slow down. Once your rate of bone turnover has stabilized at the normal level, you will begin increasing your bone mineral density as you will be building new bone.

Improvements in laboratory tests of bone resorption (bone loss) are typically seen within three to six months. Improvements in the DEXA usually take longer to manifest—one to two years.

Resources

Where Can I Find an "Integrative" Doctor Who Will Help Me Build and Keep My Bones Strong, Naturally?

To find an integrative doctor in your area, check with the organizations listed below.

- **THE ALLIANCE FOR NATURAL HEALTH USA**
  www.anh-usa.org
  1350 Connecticut Ave., NW, 5th Floor
  Washington, DC 20036
  800-230-2762
  office@anh-usa.org

- **AMERICAN ASSOCIATION OF NATUROPATHIC PHYSICIANS**
www.naturopathic.org
4435 Wisconsin Avenue, NW, Suite 403
Washington, DC 20016
202-237-8150

- **AMERICAN HOLISTIC MEDICAL ASSOCIATION**
www.holisticmedicine.org
23366 Commerce Park, Suite 101B
Beachwood, OH 44122
216-292-6644

- **AMERICAN COLLEGE FOR ADVANCEMENT IN MEDICINE**
www.acam.org
8001 Irvine Center Drive, Suite 825
Irvine, CA 92618
1-800-532-3688

- **AMERICAN ACADEMY OF ENVIRONMENTAL MEDICINE**
www.aaemonline.org
6505 E. Central Avenue, # 296
Wichita, KS 67207
316-684-5500

- **INTERNATIONAL COLLEGE OF INTEGRATIVE MEDICINE**
  www.icimed.com
  122 Thurman Street
  Box 271
  Bluffton, OH 45817
  419-358-0273

Additional Helpful Resources

- Wright, J. and L. Lenard. *Stay Young and Sexy with Bio-Identical Hormone Replacement* (Petaluma, CA: Smart Publications, 2010).

- For more information on a bone-building diet and quick, delicious recipes, visit The World's Healthiest Foods at www.whfoods.org.

Glossary

akaline phosphatase: An enzyme that is a marker for the formation of the bone-building osteoblasts.

amenorrhea: Complete loss of menstrual periods.

androgens: Male hormones.

andropause: Male menopause. Testosterone levels drop with age, resulting in insufficient production of estrogen to maintain bone.

apoptosis: Cell suicide by means of a programmed sequence of self-destruct events. Apoptosis plays a crucial role in developing and maintaining health by eliminating old cells, unnecessary cells, and unhealthy cells.

aromatase: An enzyme involved in the formation of the most potent form of estrogen.

atrial fibrillation: Irregular heartbeat.

bronchospasm: When the bands of muscle around the airways tighten uncontrollably, as in asthma.

calcaneus: Anklebone.

calcium carbonate: An alkaline form of calcium that is not as well absorbed as calcium citrate, calcium carbonate is the least expensive form of calcium and thus the form most commonly used in supplements.

calcium citrate: An acid-based and thus more bio-available form of calcium, which requires an acidic environment for absorption.

corpus luteum: Formed from the remains of the follicle after ovulation and secretes progesterone, which prepares the uterine lining for implantation of the egg, if fertilized.

creatinine: A breakdown product of creatine phosphate in muscle tissue. Higher levels indicate a decrease in kidney function and ability to excrete waste products.

C-telopeptide: Biochemical marker of bone breakdown.

cysteine: An amino acid that plays many roles in the body, one of which is as an intermediate in the methylation cycle. When levels of B_6, B_{12} and folate are inadequate, the methylation cycle stops mid-way after cysteine is converted into a harmful inflammatory product called homocysteine.

DEXA: The gold standard x-ray procedure used to evaluate bone density.

DRESS syndrome: Stands for "drug reaction with eosinophilia and systemic symptoms syndrome" and is also known as "drug hypersensitivity syndrome."

estradiol: The most potent form of estrogen.

first-degree relatives: The parents, brothers, sisters, or children.

flavin adenine dinucleotide or FAD: A coenzyme synthesized from riboflavin, FAD is required for the production of the activated forms of B_6 and folate, and also in energy metabolism, in which it acts as an electron carrier during the production of the energy currency of the body, ATP.

fragility fracture: A fracture that occurs during normal daily activities as a result of having weak, thin bones.

gastric achlorhydria: Too little stomach acid to be able to properly digest food.

gastric banding: Another surgical procedure for morbid obesity—alternative to the Roux-en-Y gastric bypass that has not been shown to produce as much bone loss as the Roux-en-Y procedure. In gastric banding, an inflatable silicone device is placed around the top portion of the stomach to create a small pouch at the top of the stomach.

gastric bypass: Surgical procedure used to treat morbid obesity, referred to in medical terminology as the Roux-en-Y procedure, greatly decreases one's ability to absorb nutrients and promotes osteoporosis.

Helicobacter pylori (H.pylori): A pathogenic bacterium that causes peptic ulcers.

hirsutism: Excessive hairiness in atypical areas, e.g., a mustache on a woman.

homocysteine: A highly inflammatory compound. High blood levels are associated with numerous chronic degenerative diseases including cardiovascular diseases and osteoporosis.

hydroxyapatite: The complex of minerals in which calcium is joined with phosphorus forming calcium phosphate, hydroxyapatite is the principal bone storage form of calcium in bone and provides its structure and strength.

hypercalcemia: Elevated blood levels of calcium.

hyperparathyroidism: Is overactivity of the parathyroid glands (hyper = excessive, above normal), resulting in excessive production of parathyroid hormone.

hyperthyroidism: A "hyperactive" thyroid.

ionized: Made to have fewer electrons.

low-energy thighbone fractures: Fractures occurring during normal daily activities.

menaquinone: Vitamin K_2, the form in which vitamin K activates osteocalcin, which pulls calcium into bone, and matrix-Gla protein, which prevents calcium from depositing in arteries.

mesenchymal stem cells: Undifferentiated cells that may develop into any one of several different types of cells, including osteoblasts, chondrocytes (cells that produce cartilage) or adipocytes (fat cells).

metformin: A patent medicine that lowers blood sugar levels and is prescribed for people with type 2 diabetes.

methionine: An essential amino acid that serves as a methyl donor in the methylation cycle (see also cysteine and homocysteine).

methylation: A cellular process involving the addition of a methyl group to a molecule, which jump starts and stops many vital processes in the body, including regulation of gene expression and protein function.

microbial biofilms: Supersized bacterial colonies that cause chronic infections, are involved in numerous diseases, and are highly resistant to antibiotics. Their likelihood of their development in the mouth, where they promote osteonecrosis of the jawbone, is increased by bisphosphonates.

myalgia: Severe muscle pain.

non-alcoholic fatty liver disease or NAFLD: Rapidly increasing liver disease, caused by insulin resistance and type 2 diabetes.

N-telopeptide: Urine or blood sample medical test that indicates the rate of bone turnover. Measures cross-linked N-telopeptides of type I collagen (NTX or NTx), a breakdown product of the type-I collagen in bone cartilage.

osteoblasts: The bone-forming cells that pull calcium, magnesium, and phosphorous from the blood to build new bone.

osteocalcin: A protein secreted by osteoblasts that plays a key role in depositing calcium in bone.

osteoclasts: Specialized bone cells that remove worn out or dead bone to make room for new bone.

osteocytes: What osteoblasts turn into after they begin secreting the bone matrix.

osteoid: A cartilage-like material into which the osteoblasts deposit calcium; also required for the cross-linking of collagen fibrils in bone, which helps to form a strong bone matrix.

osteomalacia: Bone pain.

osteonecrosis of the jaw: Jaw bone death, osteo = bone, necrosis = death.

osteopenia: Bone thinning. Accelerated bone loss, an early warning signal for developing osteoporosis.

osteoporosis: Porous bone (osteo = bone, porosis = porous)—is a progressive loss of bone that results in bone thinning and increased vulnerability to fracture.

osteoporotic fractures: Also called fragility fractures because they happen in thinned out, fragile bone.

ovulation: The release of an egg from a follicle in the ovaries.

perimenopause: The years immediately preceding menopause when levels of estrogen and progesterone begin to decline (peri=around).

periodontal ligament: The ligament that attaches the tooth to its socket in the jawbone.

phylloquinone: Vitamin K_1—type of vitamin K found in plants.

primary hyperparathyroidism: An overactive parathyroid gland whose over-activity is not caused by vitamin D deficiency.

pyridoxal-5-phosphate (P-5-P): The activated form of vitamin B_6.

resorbed: To dissolve and re-absorb.

Roux-en-Y procedure: Gastric bypass surgery in which the stomach is made smaller and part of the small intestine where many minerals and vitamins are primarily absorbed is bypassed. This causes weight loss, but also nutrient deficiencies that greatly increase risk for osteoporosis and other health problems.

sarcopenia: Loss of skeletal muscle mass, typically with aging. Sarco= flesh or muscle; penia=loss.

soluble: Able to be dissolved.

standard deviation: A statistic used as a measure of how tightly all the various participants are clustered around the mean (midline or average) in a set of data. In relation to bone loss, it signifies how much the bone mass of a specific woman differs from that of the "average" healthy 20 year old woman, the time in a woman's life when her bone mass is highest.

subtrochanter of the femur: Below the trochanter but in the upper part of the body of the thigh bone.

symptomatic hypocalcemia: A serious condition in which too little calcium is in circulation, which may result in cardiovascular collapse, very low blood pressure unresponsive to fluids and vasopressors (patent medicines that cause blood vessel constriction), and dysrhythmias (abnormal cardiac rhythms).

transverse: Crosswise.

Upper Tolerable Intake Levels (ULs): How much of a nutrient we can take daily without risk of toxicity.

venous thromboembolism: Blood clots.

Notes

1. http://en.wikipedia.org/wiki/Osteoporosis.

2. Riggs, B. L., L. J. Melton 3rd, R. A. Robb, et al. 2004. Population-based study of age and sex differences in bone volumetric density, size, geometry, and structure at different skeletal sites. *J Bone Miner Res* 19:1945–54. PMID: 15537436.

3. Bilezikian, J. P. 1999. Osteoporosis in men. *J Clin Endocrinol Metab* Oct.; 84(10):3431–4. PMID: 10522975.

4. Nochowitz, B. 2009. An update on osteoporosis. *Am J Ther* Sept-Oct;16(5):437–445. PMID: 19262365.

5. Binkley, N. 2006. Osteoporosis in men. *Arq Bras Endocrinol Metab* 50/4:764–774. PMID: 17117301.

    Stock, H., A. Schneider, and E. Strauss. 2004. Osteoporosis: a disease in men. *Clin Orthop Relat Res* Aug;(425):143–51. PMID: 15292799.

6. Center, J. R., T. V. Nguyen, D. Schneider, et al. 1999. Mortality after all major types of osteoporotic fracture in men and women: an observational study. *Lancet* 353:878–82. PMID: 10093980.

   Pande, I., D. L. Scott, T. W. O'Neill, et al. 2006. Quality of life, morbidity, and mortality after low trauma hip fracture in men. *Ann Rheum Dis* 65:87–92. PMID: 16079173.

7. Null, G., D. Rasio, and C. Dean. *Death by Medicine* (Mt. Jackson, VA: Praktikos Books, 2010).

8. American Association of Poison Control Centers. 2008 Report, http://www.aapcc.org/dnn/Portals/0/2008annualreport.pdf (accessed 6-2-2010).

9. http://www.fda.gov/cder/drug/infopage/bisphosphonates/default.htm

10. Odvina, C.V., J. E. Zerwekh, D. S. Rao, et al. 2005. Severely suppressed bone turnover: a potential complication of alendronate therapy. *J Clin Endocrinol Metab* Mar;90(3):1294–301. PMID: 15598694.

11. Document #4, Judge Daubert ruling. "Opinion and 6 Order", from Judge John F Keenan, United States District Court, Southern District of New York, Case 1:06-md-01789-JFK-JCF. Document 750 filed 07/27/2009: pages 21, 36, 45.

12. Favia, G., G. P. Pilolli, E. Maiorano. 2009. Osteonecrosis of the jaw correlated to bisphosphonate therapy in non-oncologic patients: clinicopathological features of 24 patients. *J Rheumatol* Dec;36(12):2780–7. PMID: 19884275.

13. Lo, J. C., F. S. O'Ryan, N. P. Gordon, et al. 2009. Prevalence of osteonecrosis of the jaw in patients with oral bisphosphonate exposure. *J Oral Maxillofac Surg* Jun 30. PMID: 19772941.

14. Favia, G., G. P. Pilolli, and E. Maiorano. 2009. Osteonecrosis of the jaw correlated to bisphosphonate therapy in non-oncologic patients: clinicopathological features of 24 patients. *J Rheumatol* Dec;36(12):2780–7. PMID: 19884275.

   Palaska, P. K., V. Cartsos, and A. I. Zavras. 2009. Bisphosphonates and time to osteonecrosis development. *Oncologist* Nov;14(11):1154–66. PMID: 19897878.

   Marx, R. E. 2008. Bisphosphonate-induced osteonecrosis of the jaws: a challenge, a responsibility, and an opportunity. *Int J Periodontics Restorative Dent* Feb;28(1):5–6. PMID: 18351197.

   Rogers, S., N. Rahman, and D. Ryan. 2010. Guidelines for treating patients taking bisphosphonates prior to dental extractions. *J Ir Dent Assoc* Feb-Mar;56(1):40. PMID: 20337145.

   Dello Russo, N. M., M. K. Jeffcoat, R. E. Marx, et al. 2007. Osteonecrosis in the jaws of patients who are using oral biphosphonates to treat osteoporosis. *Int J Oral Maxillofac Implants* Jan-Feb;22(1):146–53. PMID: 17340909.

   Lee, J. 2009. Complication related to bisphosphonate therapy: osteonecrosis of the jaw. *J Infus Nurs* Nov-Dec;32(6):330–5. PMID: 19918142.

Lo, J. C., F. S. O'Ryan, N. P. Gordon, et al. 2010. Prevalence of osteonecrosis of the jaw in patients with oral bisphosphonate exposure. *J Oral Maxillofac Surg* Feb;68(2):243–53. PMID: 19772941.

Longo, R., M. A. Castellana, and G. Gasparini. 2009. Bisphosphonate-related osteonecrosis of the jaw and left thumb. *J Clin Oncol* Dec 10;27(35):e242–3. PMID: 19858386.

Kyrgidis, A. and E. Verrou. 2010. Fatigue in bone: a novel phenomenon attributable to bisphosphonate use. *Bone* Feb;46(2):556; author reply 557–8. Epub 2009 Sep 29. PMID: 19796720.

Vassiliou, V., N. Tselis, and D. Kardamakis. 2010. Osteonecrosis of the Jaws: Clinicopathologic and Radiologic Characteristics, Preventive and Therapeutic Strategies. *Strahlenther Onkol* Apr 26. [Epub ahead of print] PMID: 20437019.

Kyrgidis, A. and K. Vahtsevanos. 2010. Bisphosphonate-related osteonecrosis of the jaws: A review of 34 cases and evaluation of risk. *J Craniomaxillofac Surg* Apr 29. [Epub ahead of print] PMID: 20434920.

Assael, L. A. 2009. Oral bisphosphonates as a cause of bisphosphonate-related osteonecrosis of the jaws: clinical findings, assessment of risks, and preventive strategies. *J Oral Maxillofac Surg* May;67(5 Suppl):35–43. PMID: 19371813.

Migliorati, C. A., K. Mattos, and M. J. Palazzolo. 2010. How patients' lack of knowledge about oral bisphosphonates can interfere with medical and dental care. *J Am Dent Assoc* May;141(5):562–6. PMID: 20436104.

Filleul,O., E. Crompot and S. Saussez. 2010. Bisphosphonate-induced osteonecrosis of the jaw: a review of 2,400 patient cases. *J Cancer Res Clin Oncol* Aug;136(8):1117-24. Epub 2010 May 28. PMID: 20508948.

Sarin, J., S. S. DeRossi and S. O. Akintoye. 2008. Updates on bisphosphonates and potential pathobiology of bisphosphonate-induced jaw osteonecrosis. *Oral Dis* Apr;14(3):277-85. PMID: 18336375.

15. Favia, G., G. P. Pilolli, and E. Maiorano. 2009. Histologic and histomorphometric features of bisphosphonate-related osteonecrosis of the jaws: an analysis of 31 cases with confocal laser scanning microscopy. *Bone* Sep;45(3):406–13. Epub 2009 May 18. PMID: 19450715.

Stepan, J. J., D. B. Burr, I. Pavo, et al. 2007. Low bone mineral density is associated with bone microdamage accumulation in postmenopausal women with osteoporosis. *Bone* Sep;41(3):378–85. PMID: 17597017.

16. Sedghizadeh, P. P., K. Stanley, M. Caligiuri, S. Hofkes, B. Lowry, and C. F. Shuler. 2009. Oral bisphosphonate use and the prevalence of osteonecrosis of the jaw: An institutional inquiry. *J Am Dent Assoc* 40:61–66. PMID: 19119168.

Sedghizadeh, P. P., S. K. Kumar, A. Gorur, et al. 2008. Identification of microbial biofilms in osteonecrosis of the jaws secondary to bisphosphonate therapy. *J Oral Maxillofac Surg* Apr;66(4):767–75. PMID: 18355603.

17. Pazianas, M., P. Miller, W. A. Blumentals, et al. 2007. A review of the literature on osteonecrosis of the jaw in patients with osteoporosis treated with oral bisphosphonates: prevalence, risk factors, and clinical characteristics. *Clin Ther* Aug;29(8):1548–58. PMID: 17919538.

18. Edwards, B. J., J. W. Hellstein, P. L. Jacobsen, et al. 2008. Updated recommendations for managing the care of patients receiving oral bisphosphonate therapy: an advisory statement from the American Dental Association Council on Scientific Affairs. *J Am Dent Assoc* Dec;139(12):1674–7. PMID: 19047674. http://www.ada.org/prof/resources/topics/osteonecrosis.asp.

19. Parker Waichman Alonso LLP. Breaking News. Osteonecrosis of the Jaw, http://www.yourlawyer.com/topics/overview/osteonecrosis_of_the_jaw_onj/.

Arrain, Y. and T. Masud. 2009. Bisphosphonates and osteonecrosis of the jaw—current thoughts. *Dent Update* Sep;36(7):415–9. PMID: 19810397.

20. Estefanía Fresco, R., R. Ponte Fernández, J. M. Aguirre Urizar. 2006. Bisphosphonates and oral pathology II. Osteonecrosis of the jaws: review of the literature before 2005. *Med Oral Patol Oral Cir Bucal* Nov 1;11(6):E456–61. PMID: 17072246.

21. Kumar, S. K., M. Meru, and P. Sedghizadeh. 2008. Osteonecrosis of the jaws secondary to

bisphosphonate therapy: a case series. *J Contemp Dent Pract* Jan 1;9(1):63–9. PMID: 18176650.

22. Sedghizadeh, P. P., S. K. Kumar, A. Gorur, et al. 2008. Identification of microbial biofilms in osteonecrosis of the jaws secondary to bisphosphonate therapy. *J Oral Maxillofac Surg* Apr;66(4):767–75. PMID: 18355603.

23. Mak, A., M. W. Cheung, R. C. Ho, et al. 2009. Bisphosphonates and atrial fibrillation: Bayesian meta-analyses of randomized controlled trials and observational studies. *BMC Musculoskelet Disord* Sep 21;10:113. PMID: 19772579.

Bhuriya, R., M. Singh, J. Molnar, et al. 2010. Bisphosphonate use in women and the risk of atrial fibrillation: A systematic review and meta-analysis. *Int J Cardiol* Jan 3. [Epub ahead of print] PMID: 20051297.

24. Naccarelli. G., A. Capucci, C. Lau, and O. Oseroff. Identifying atrial fibrillation-preventing stroke. On-line medical seminar. November 13, 2010, http://www.theheart.org/article/1020235.do.

Lopes, R. D., J. P. Piccini, E. M. Hylek, et al. 2008. Antithrombotic therapy in atrial fibrillation: guidelines translated for the clinician. *J Thromb Thrombolysis* Dec;26(3):167–74. PMID: 18807225.

25. Cummings, S. R., A. V. Schwartz, et al. 2007. Alendronate and atrial fibrillation. *N Engl J Med* May 3;356(18):1895–6. PMID: 17476024.

26. Huang, W. F., Y. W. Tsai, Y. W. Wen, et al. 2009. Osteoporosis treatment and atrial fibrillation: alendronate versus raloxifene. *Menopause* Aug 12. [Epub ahead of print] PMID: 19680161.

27. Heckbert, S. R., G. Li, S. R. Cummings, et al. 2008. Use of alendronate and risk of incident atrial fibrillation in women. *Arch Intern Med* Apr 28;168(8):826–31. PMID: 18443257.

28. Papapetrou, P. D. 2009. Bisphosphonate-associated adverse events. *Hormones* (Athens) Apr-Jun;8(2):96–110. PMID: 19570737.

29. Woo, C., G. Gao, S. Wade, et al. 2010. Gastrointestinal side effects in postmenopausal women using osteoporosis therapy: 1-year findings in the POSSIBLE US study. *Curr Med Res Opin* Apr;26(4):1003–9. PMID: 20201623.

30. Green, J., G. Czanner, G. Reeves, et al. 2010. Oral bisphosphonates and risk of cancer of oesophagus, stomach, and colorectum: case-control analysis within a UK primary care cohort. *BMJ* Sep 1;341:c4444. doi: 10.1136/bmj.c4444. PMID: 20813820.

31. Body, J. J. 2001. Dosing regimens and main adverse events of bisphosphonates. *Semin Oncol* Aug;28(4 Suppl 11):49–53. PMID: 11544576.

32. Merck Sharp & Dohme (New Zealand). Limited. Fosamax (alendronate) data sheet, 17 October 2005, http://www.medsafe.govt.nz/profs/Datasheet/f/Fosamaxtab.htm.

33. Mazj, S. and S. M. Lichtman. 2004. Renal dysfunction associated with bisphosphonate use: Retrospective analysis of 293 patients with respect to age and other clinical characteristics. *Journal of Clinical Oncology* ASCO Annual Meeting Proceedings (Post-Meeting Edition). Vol 22, No 14S (July 15 Supplement), 8039, available at http://meeting.ascopubs.org/cgi/content/abstract/22/14_suppl/8039 (accessed 6-18-10).

Diel, I. J., R. Weide, H. Köppler, et al. 2009. Risk of renal impairment after treatment with ibandronate versus zoledronic acid: a retrospective medical records review. *Support Care Cancer* Jun;17(6):719–25. Epub 2008 Dec 17. PMID: 19089462.

34. Perman, M. J., A. W. Lucky, J. E. Heubi, et al. 2009. Severe symptomatic hypocalcemia in a patient with RDEB treated with intravenous zoledronic acid. *Arch Dermatol* Jan;145(1):95–6. PMID: 19153360.

Mishra, A. 2008. Symptomatic hypocalcemia following intravenous administration of zoledronic acid in a breast cancer patient. *J Postgrad Med* Jul-Sep;54(3):237. PMID: 18626181.

Chennuru, S., J. Koduri, M. A. Baumann. 2008. Risk factors for symptomatic hypocalcaemia complicating treatment with zoledronic acid. *Intern Med J* Aug;38(8):635–7. Epub 2008 Feb 17. PMID: 18284458.

Aksoy, S., H. Abali, M. Dinçer, et al. 2004. Hypocalcemic effect of zoledronic acid or other bisphosphonates may contribute to their antiangiogenic properties. *Med Hypotheses* 62(6):942–4. PMID: 15142653.

Tanvetyanon, T. and A. M. Choudhury. 2004. Hypocalcemia and azotemia associated with zoledronic acid and interferon alfa. *Ann Pharmacother* Mar;38(3):418–21. PMID: 14970365.

35. Kyrgidis, A. and E. Verrou. 2009. Fatigue in bone: A novel phenomenon attributable to bisphosphonate use. *Bone* Sep 29.PMID: 19796720.

36. Odvina, C.V., J. E. Zerwekh, D. S. Rao, et al. 2005. Severely suppressed bone turnover: a potential complication of alendronate therapy. *J Clin Endocrinol Metab* Mar;90(3):1294–301. PMID: 15598694.

37. Goh, S. K., K.Y. Yang, J. S. Koh, et al. 2007. Subtrochanteric insufficiency fractures in patients on alendronate therapy: a caution. *J Bone Joint Surg Br* 89(3):349–353. PMID: 17356148.

38. Nevasier, A.S., J. M. Lane, B. A. Lenart, et al. 2008. Low-energy femoral shaft fractures associated with alendronate use. *J Orthop Trauma* 22(5):346–350. PMID: 18448990.

39. Stepan, J. J., D. B. Burr, I. Pavo, et al. 2007. Low bone mineral density is associated with bone microdamage accumulation in postmenopausal women with osteoporosis. *Bone* Sep;41(3):378–85. PMID: 17597017.

40. Ing-Lorenzini, K., J. Desmeules, O. Plachta, et al. 2009. Low-energy femoral fractures associated

with the long-term use of bisphosphonates: a case series from a Swiss university hospital. *Drug Saf* 32(9):775–85. PMID: 19670917.

41. Watters, C. 2010. Bisphosphonate Therapy for Osteoporosis: A Potential Risk for Subtrochanteric Fractures. *Orthopaedic Nursing* 29(3):210-213, May/June doi: 10.1097/ NOR.0b013e3181db5485.

    Bamrungsong, T. and C. Pongchaiyakul. 2010. Bilateral atypical femoral fractures after long-term alendronate therapy: a case report. *J Med Assoc Thai* May;93(5):620-4. PMID: 20524451.

    Abrahamsen, B. 2010. Adverse effects of bisphosphonates. *Calcif Tissue Int* Jun;86(6):421-35. Epub 2010 Apr 21. PMID: 20407762.

    Giusti, A., N. A. Hamdy and S. E. Papapoulos. 2010. Atypical fractures of the femur and bisphosphonate therapy: A systematic review of case/case series studies. *Bone* Aug;47(2):169-80. Epub 2010 May 20. PMID: 20493982.

    Girgis, C. M. and M. J. Seibel. 2010. Atypical femur fractures: a complication of prolonged bisphosphonate therapy? *Med J Aust* Aug 16;193(4):196-8. PMID: 20712536.

42. Benhamou, C. L. 2007. Effects of osteoporosis medications on bone quality. *Joint Bone Spine* Jan;74(1):39-47. PMID: 17196423.

    Capeci, C. M. and N. C. Tejwani. 2009. Bilateral low-energy simultaneous or sequential femoral fractures in patients on long-term alendronate therapy. *J Bone Joint Surg Am* Nov;91(11):2556–61. PMID: 19884427.

Schneider, J. P. 2009. Bisphosphonates and low-impact femoral fractures: current evidence on alendronate-fracture risk. *Geriatrics* Jan;64(1):18–23. PMID: 19256578.

Bunning, R.D., R. J. Rentfro and J. S. Jelinek. 2010. Low-energy femoral fractures associated with long-term bisphosphonate use in a rehabilitation setting: a case series. *PM R* Jan;2(1):76–80. PMID: 20129517.

Schilcher, J. and P. Aspenberg. 2009. Incidence of stress fractures of the femoral shaft in women treated with bisphosphonate. *Acta Orthop* Aug;80(4):413–5. PMID: 19568963.

Lenart, B. A., A. S. Neviaser, S. Lyman, et al. 2009. Association of low-energy femoral fractures with prolonged bisphosphonate use: a case control study. *Osteoporos Int* Aug;20(8):1353–62. Epub 2008 Dec 9. PMID: 19066707.

Goddard, M. S., K. R. Reid, J. C. Johnston, et al. 2009. Atraumatic bilateral femur fracture in long-term bisphosphonate use. *Orthopedics* Aug;32(8). PMID: 19708622.

Capeci, C. M. and N. C. Tejwani. 2009. Bilateral low-energy simultaneous or sequential femoral fractures in patients on long-term alendronate therapy. *J Bone Joint Surg Am* Nov;91(11):2556–61. PMID: 19884427.

43. Yamaguchi, T. and T. Sugimoto. 2009. [New development in bisphosphonate treatment. When and how long should patients take bisphosphonates for osteoporosis?] *Clin Calcium* Jan;19(1):38–43. PMID: 19122263.

44. Romo, C. and L. Salahi. Fosamax: Is Long Term Use of Bone Strengthening Drug Linked to Fractures? ABC News, March 8, 2010, http://abcnews. go.com/WN/WorldNews/osteoporosis-drugs-fosamax-increase-risk-broken-bones-women/ story?id=10044066.

Romo, C., L. Salahi and D. Childs. FDA to Investigate Possible Osteoporosis Drug-Femur Fracture Link After ABC News Report. ABC News, March 10, 2010, http://abcnews.go.com/WN/WellnessNews/ fda-consult-experts-fracture-risk-bone-drugs/ story?id=10065341.

FDA Drug Safety Communication: Ongoing safety review of oral bisphosphonates and atypical subtrochanteric femur fractures. http://www.fda.gov/Drugs/DrugSafety/ PostmarketDrugSafetyInformationforPatient-sandProviders/ucm203891.htm.

45. FDA Drug Safety Communication. http://www. fda.gov/Drugs/DrugSafety/ucm229009.htm.

FDA Consumer Update. http://www.fda.gov/ ForConsumers/ConsumerUpdates/ucm229127. htm.

46. Solomon, D.H., M. C. Hochberg, H. Mogun, et al. 2009. The relation between bisphosphonate use

and non-union of fractures of the humerus in older adults. *Osteoporos Int* Jun;20(6):895–901. Epub 2008 Oct 9. PMID: 18843515.

47. Knight, R. J., C. Reddy, M. A. Rtshiladze, et al. 2010. Bisphosphonate-related osteonecrosis of the jaw: tip of the iceberg. *J Craniofac Surg* Jan;21(1):25–32. Review. PMID: 20072026.

48. Prommer, E. E. 2009. Toxicity of bisphosphonates. *J Palliat Med* Nov;12(11):1061–5. PMID: 19922007.

    Kyrgidis, A., S. Triaridis, K. Vahtsevanos, et al. 2009. Osteonecrosis of the jaw and bisphosphonate use in breast cancer patients. *Expert Rev Anticancer Ther* Aug;9(8):1125–34. PMID: 19671032.

    Gebara, S. N. and H. Moubayed. 2009. Risk of osteonecrosis of the jaw in cancer patients taking bisphosphonates. *Am J Health Syst Pharm* Sep 1;66(17):1541–7. PMID: 19710437.

49. Ferran, L. and K. McKarthy. New Weapon in Breast Cancer Battle? Experts Cautious. Dec. 11, 2009, http://abcnews.go.com/.

50. Body, J. J. 2008. [Update on treatment of postmenopausal osteoporosis] *Rev Med Brux* Sep;29(4):301–9. PMID: 18949981.

    Valverde, P. 2008. Pharmacotherapies to manage bone loss-associated diseases: a quest for the perfect benefit-to-risk ratio. *Curr Med Chem* 15(3):284–304. Review. PMID: 18288984.

Uebelhart, D., D. Frey, P. Frey-Rindova, et al. 2003. [Therapy of osteoporosis: bisphosphonates, SERM's, teriparatide and strontium] *Z Rheumatol* Dec;62(6):512–7. Review. PMID: 14685711.

O'Donnell, S., A. Cranney, G. A. Wells, et al. 2006. Strontium ranelate for preventing and treating postmenopausal osteoporosis. *Cochrane Database Syst Rev* Oct 18;(4):CD005326. PMID: 17054253.

Stevenson, M., S. Davis, M. Lloyd-Jones, et al. 2007. The clinical effectiveness and cost-effectiveness of strontium ranelate for the prevention of osteoporotic fragility fractures in postmenopausal women. *Health Technol Assess* Feb;11(4):1–134. PMID: 17280622.

Reginster, J. Y., R. Deroisy and I. Jupsin. 2003. Strontium ranelate: a new paradigm in the treatment of osteoporosis. *Drugs Today* (Barc) Feb;39(2):89–101. PMID: 12698204.

51. Ma, J., R. A. Johns and R. S. Stafford. 2007. Americans are not meeting current calcium recommendations. *Am J Clin Nutr* May;85(5):1361–6. PMID: 17490974.

52. Hale, G.E. and H. G. Burger. 2009. Hormonal changes and biomarkers in late reproductive age, menopausal transition and menopause. *Best Pract Res Clin Obstet Gynaecol* Feb;23(1):7–23. PMID: 19046657.

53. Binkley, N. 2006. Osteoporosis in men. *Arq Bras Endocrinol Metabol* Aug;50(4):764–74. PMID: 17117301.

Tuck, S. P. and R. M. Francis. 2009. Testosterone, bone and osteoporosis. *Front Horm Res* 37:123–32. PMID: 19011293.

54. Ross, R. W. and E. J. Small. 2002. Osteoporosis in men treated with androgen deprivation therapy for prostate cancer. *J Urol* May;167(5):1952–6. PMID: 11956415.

55. Grossman, M. I., J. B. Kirsner and I. E. Gillespie. 1963. Basal and histalog-stimulated gastric secretion in control subjects and in patients with peptic ulcer or gastric cancer. *Gastroenterology* Jul;45:14–26. PMID: 14046306.

56. Nicar, M. J. and C. Y. Pak. 1985. Calcium bioavailability from calcium carbonate and calcium citrate. *J Clin Endocrinol Metab* Aug;61(2):391–3. PMID: 4008614.

Wood, R. J. and C. Serfaty-Lacrosniere. 1992. Gastric acidity, atrophic gastritis, and calcium absorption. *Nutr Rev* Feb;50(2):33–40. PMID: 1570081.

57. Nicar, M. J. and C. Y. Pak. 1985. Calcium bioavailability from calcium carbonate and calcium citrate. *J Clin Endocrinol Metab* Aug;61(2):391–3. PMID: 4008614.

Wood, R. J. and C. Serfaty-Lacrosniere. 1992. Gastric acidity, atrophic gastritis, and calcium absorption. *Nutr Rev* Feb;50(2):33–40. PMID: 1570081.

58. Hanzlik, R.P., S. C. Fowler and D. H. Fisher. 2005. Relative bioavailability of calcium from calcium

formate, calcium citrate, and calcium carbonate. *J Pharmacol Exp Ther* Jun;313(3):1217–22. PMID: 15734899.

Reinwald, S., C. M. Weaver and J. J. Kester. 2008. The health benefits of calcium citrate malate: a review of the supporting science. *Adv Food Nutr Res* 54:219–346. PMID: 18291308.

Tondapu, P., D. Provost, B. Adams-Huet, et al. 2009. Comparison of the absorption of calcium carbonate and calcium citrate after Roux-en-Y gastric bypass. *Obes Surg* Sep;19(9):1256–61. PMID: 19437082.

59. Straub, D. A. 2007. Calcium supplementation in clinical practice: a review of forms, doses, and indications. *Nutr Clin Pract* Jun;22(3):286–96. PMID: 17507729.

60. Licata, A. A., E. Bou, F. C. Bartter, et al. 1981. Acute effects of dietary protein on calcium metabolism in patients with osteoporosis. *J Gerontol* Jan;36(1):14–9. PMID: 7451829.

61. New, S. A. 2004. Do vegetarians have a normal bone mass? *Osteoporos Int* Sep;15(9):679–88. PMID: 15258721.

Marsh, A. G., T. V. Sanchez, F. L. Chaffee, et al. 1983. Bone mineral mass in adult lacto-ovo-vegetarian and omnivorous males. *Am J Clin Nutr* Mar;37(3):453–6. PMID: 6687507.

Cooper, C., E. J. Atkinson, D. D. Hensrud, et al. 1996. Dietary protein intake and bone mass in women. *Calcif Tissue Int* May;58(5):320–5. PMID: 8661965.

62. Fulgoni, V. L. 3rd. 2008. Current protein intake in America: analysis of the National Health and Nutrition Examination Survey, 2003–2004. *Am J Clin Nutr* May;87(5):1554S-1557S. PMID: 18469286.

63. Kerstetter, J. E., K. O. O'Brien and K. L. Insogna. 2003. Low protein intake: the impact on calcium and bone homeostasis in humans. *J Nutr* Mar;133(3):855S-861S. PMID: 12612169.

64. Kerstetter, J. E., K. O. O'Brien and K. L. Insogna. 2003. Dietary protein, calcium metabolism, and skeletal homeostasis revisited. *Am J Clin Nutr* Sep;78(3 Suppl):584S-592S. PMID: 12936953.

65. Pizzorno, J. E. and M. T. Murray eds. *Textbook of Natural Medicine*, 3rd Ed. Vol. 2, (St Louis, MO: Elsevier, 2006), p. 1982.

   Gross, L. S., L. Li, E. S. Ford and S. Liu. 2004. Increased consumption of refined carbohydrates and the epidemic of type 2 diabetes in the United States: an ecologic assessment. *Am J Clin Nutr* May;79(5):774–9. PMID: 15113714.

66. Olshansky, S. J., D. J. Passaro, R. C. Hershow, et al. 2005. A potential decline in life expectancy in the United States in the 21st century. *N Engl J Med* Mar 17;352(11):1138–45. PMID: 15784668.

67. Pizzorno, J. E. and M. T. Murray eds. *Textbook of Natural Medicine*, 3rd Ed. Vol. 2, (St Louis, MO: Elsevier, 2006), p. 1982.

68. Byers, T. 1993. Dietary trends in the United States. Relevance to cancer prevention. *Cancer* Aug 1;72(3 Suppl):1015–8. PMID: 8334652.

69. Block, G. 1991. Dietary guidelines and the results of food consumption surveys. *Am J Clin Nutr* Jan;53(1 Suppl):356S-357S. PMID: 1985410.

70. Saito, M. 2009. [Biochemical markers of bone turnover. New aspect. Bone collagen metabolism: new biological markers for estimation of bone quality] *Clin Calcium* Aug;19(8):1110-7. PMID: 19638694.

Petramala, L., M. Acca, C. M. Francucci, et al. 2009. Hyperhomocysteinemia: a biochemical link between bone and cardiovascular system diseases? *J Endocrinol Invest* 32(4 Suppl):10-4. PMID: 19724160.

Yilmaz, N. and E. Eren. 2009. Homocysteine oxidative stress and relation to bone mineral density in postmenopausal osteoporosis. *Aging Clin Exp Res* Aug-Oct;21(4-5):353-7. PMID: 19959926.

Haliloglu, B., F. B. Aksungar, E. Ilter, et al. 2010. Relationship between bone mineral density, bone turnover markers and homocysteine, folate and vitamin B12 levels in postmenopausal women. *Arch Gynecol Obstet* Apr;281(4):663-8. Epub 2009 Nov 28. PMID: 19946695.

Leboff, M. S., R. Narweker, A. LaCroix, et al. 2009. *J Clin Endocrinol Metab* Apr;94(4):1207-13. PMID: 19174498.

71. Andreotti, F., F. Burzotta, A. Manzoli, et al. 2000. Homocysteine and risk of cardiovascular disease. *J Thromb Thrombolysis* Jan;9(1):13-21. PMID: 10590184.

72. Stanger, O., B. Fowler, K. Piertzik, et al. 2009. Homocysteine, folate and vitamin B12 in neuropsychiatric diseases: review and treatment recommendations. *Expert Rev Neurother* Sep;9(9):1393–412. PMID: 19769453.

73. Ferechide, D. and D. Radulescu. 2009. Hyperhomocysteinemia in renal diseases. *J Med Life* Jan-Mar;2(1):53–9. PMID: 20108491.

Zoccali, C. 2005. Biomarkers in chronic kidney disease: utility and issues towards better understanding. *Curr Opin Nephrol Hypertens* Nov;14(6):532–7. PMID: 16205471.

Ingrosso, D., A. F. Perna. 2009. Epigenetics in hyperhomocysteinemic states. A special focus on uremia. *Biochim Biophys Acta* Sep;1790(9):892–9. PMID: 19245874.

Righetti, M. 2009. Protective effect of vitamin B therapy on bone and cardiovascular disease. *Recent Pat Cardiovasc Drug Discov* Jan;4(1):37–44. PMID: 19149705.

Trimarchi, H., P. Young, M. L. Díaz, et al. 2005. [Hyperhomocysteinemia as a vascular risk factor in chronic hemodialysis patients] *Medicina* (B Aires) 65(6):513–7. PMID: 16433478.

74. Woolf, K., M. M. Manore. 2008. Elevated plasma homocysteine and low vitamin B-6 status in non-supplementing older women with rheumatoid arthritis. *J Am Diet Assoc* Mar;108(3):443–53; discussion 454. PMID: 18313425.

75. Wile, D. J. and C. Toth. 2010. Association of metformin, elevated homocysteine, and methylmalonic acid levels and clinically worsened diabetic peripheral neuropathy. *Diabetes Care.* 2010 Jan;33(1):156–61. Epub 2009 Oct 21. PMID: 19846797.

Pflipsen, M. C., R. C. Oh, A. Saguil, et al. 2009. The prevalence of vitamin B(12) deficiency in patients with type 2 diabetes: a cross-sectional study. *J Am Board Fam Med* Sep-Oct;22(5):528–34. PMID: 19734399.

76. Shah, S., R. J. Bell, S. R. Davis. 2006. Homocysteine, estrogen and cognitive decline. *Climacteric* Apr;9(2):77–87. PMID: 16698655.

Sultan, N., M. A. Khan and S. Malik. 2007. Effect of folic acid supplementation on homocysteine level in postmenopausal women. *J Ayub Med Coll Abbottabad* Oct-Dec;19(4):78–81. PMID: 18693605.

77. McLean, R. R., P. F. Jacques, J. Selhub, et al. 2008. Plasma B vitamins, homocysteine, and their relation with bone loss and hip fracture in elderly men and women. *J Clin Endocrinol Metab* Jun;93(6):2206–12. PMID: 18364381.

78. Lussana, F., M. L. Zighetti, P. Bucciarelli, et al. 2003. Blood levels of homocysteine, folate, vitamin B_6 and B12 in women using oral contraceptives compared to non-users. *Thromb Res* 112(1–2):37–41. PMID: 15013271.

79. Pfeiffer, C. M., S. P. Caudill, E. W. Gunter, et al. 2005. Biochemical indicators of B vitamin status

in the US population after folic acid fortification: results from the National Health and Nutrition Examination Survey 1999–2000. *Am J Clin Nutr* Aug;82(2):442–50. PMID: 16087991.

80. Pennypacker, L. C., R. H. Allen, et al. 1992. High prevalence of cobalamin deficiency in elderly out-patients. *J Am Geriatr Soc* Dec;40(12):1197–204. PMID: 1447433.

81. Allen, L. H. 2009. How common is vitamin B-12 deficiency? *Am J Clin Nutr* Feb;89(2):693S-6S. Epub 2008 Dec 30. PMID: 19116323.

82. Pflipsen, M. C., R. C. Oh, A. Saguil, et al. 2009. The prevalence of vitamin B(12) deficiency in patients with type 2 diabetes: a cross-sectional study. *J Am Board Fam Med* Sep-Oct;22(5):528–34. PMID: 19734399.

83. Fain, O. 2005. Musculoskeletal manifestations of scurvy. *Joint Bone Spine* Mar;72(2):124–8. PMID: 15797491.

Hall, S. L. and G. A. Greendale. 1998. The relation of dietary vitamin C intake to bone mineral density: results from the PEPI study. *Calcif Tissue Int* Sep;63(3):183–9. PMID: 9701620.

84. Sahni, S., M. T. Hannan, D. Gagnon, et al. 2009. Protective effect of total and supplemental vitamin C intake on the risk of hip fracture—a 17-year follow-up from the Framingham Osteoporosis Study. *Osteoporos Int* Nov;20(11):1853–61. PMID: 19347239.

85. Martínez-Ramírez, M. J., S. Palma Pérez, A. D. Delgado-Martínez, et al. 2007. Vitamin C, vitamin B12, folate and the risk of osteoporotic fractures. A case-control study. *Int J Vitam Nutr Res* Nov;77(6):359–68. PMID: 18622945.

86. Pasco, J. A., M. J. Henry, L. K. Wilkinson, et al. 2006. Antioxidant vitamin supplements and markers of bone turnover in a community sample of nonsmoking women. *J Womens Health* (Larchmt) Apr;15(3):295–300. PMID: 16620188.

87. Schleicher, R. L., M. D. Carroll, E. S. Ford, et al. 2009. Serum vitamin C and the prevalence of vitamin C deficiency in the United States: 2003–2004 National Health and Nutrition Examination Survey (NHANES). *Am J Clin Nutr* Nov;90(5):1252–63 PMID: 19675106.

88. Palacios, C. 2006. The role of nutrients in bone health, from A to Z. *Crit Rev Food Sci Nutr* 46(8):621–8. PMID: 17092827.

 Morton, D. J., E. L. Barrett-Connor and D. L. Schneider. 2001. Vitamin C supplement use and bone mineral density in postmenopausal women. *J Bone Miner Res* Jan;16(1):135–40. PMID: 11149477.

89. Pizzorno, J. E. *Total Wellness* (Rocklin, CA: Prima Publishing, 1996), p. 44–45, 62.

90. Schleicher, R. L., M. D. Carroll, E. S. Ford, et al. 2009. Serum vitamin C and the prevalence of vitamin C deficiency in the United States: 2003–2004 National Health and Nutrition

Examination Survey (NHANES). *Am J Clin Nutr* Nov;90(5):1252–63 PMID: 19675106.

91. Lazcano-Ponce, E., J. Tamayo, R. Díaz, et al. 2009. Correlation trends for bone mineral density in Mexican women: evidence of familiar predisposition. *Salud Publica Mex* 51 Suppl 1:s93–9. PMID: 19287898

92. Pizzorno, J. E. and M. T. Murray, "Osteoporosis", in *Textbook of Natural Medicine*, 3rd ed., (St. Louis: Elsevier, 2006), Ch. 196, 2:1978.

93. Makovey, J., T. V. Nguyen, V. Naganathan, et al. 2007. Genetic effects on bone loss in peri- and postmenopausal women: a longitudinal twin study. *J Bone Miner Res* Nov;22(11):1773–80. PMID: 17620052.

    Sigurdsson, G., B. V. Halldorsson, U. Styrkarsdottir, et al. 2008. Impact of genetics on low bone mass in adults. *J Bone Miner Res* Oct;23(10):1584–90. PMID: 18505373.

    Zhai, G., T. Andrew, B. S. Kato, et al. 2009. Genetic and environmental determinants on bone loss in postmenopausal Caucasian women: a 14-year longitudinal twin study. *Osteoporos Int* Jun;20(6):949–53. PMID: 18810303.

94. Valderas, J. P., S. Velasco, S. Solari, et al. 2009. Increase of bone resorption and the parathyroid hormone in postmenopausal women in the long-term after Roux-en-Y gastric bypass. *Obes Surg* Aug;19(8):1132–8. Epub 2009 Jun 11. PMID: 19517199.

De Prisco, C. and S. N. Levine. 2005. Metabolic bone disease after gastric bypass surgery for obesity. *Am J Med Sci* Feb;329(2):57–61. PMID: 15711420.

95. Tice, J. A., L. Karliner, J. Walsh, et al. 2008. Gastric banding or bypass? A systematic review comparing the two most popular bariatric procedures. *Am J Med* Oct;121(10):885–93. PMID: 18823860.

96. Wang, A. and A. Powell. 2009. The effects of obesity surgery on bone metabolism: what orthopedic surgeons need to know. *Am J Orthop* (Belle Mead NJ) Feb;38(2):77–9. PMID: 19340369.

97. Goode, L. R., R. E. Brolin, H. A. Chowdhury, et al. 2004. Bone and gastric bypass surgery: effects of dietary calcium and vitamin D. *Obes Res* Jan;12(1):40–7. PMID: 14742841.

98. Nakchbandi, I. A., S. W. van der Merwe. 2009. Current understanding of osteoporosis associated with liver disease. *Nat Rev Gastroenterol Hepatol* Nov;6(11):660–70. PMID: 19881518.

Jean, G., J. C. Terrat, T. Vanel, et al. 2008. Daily oral 25-hydroxycholecalciferol supplementation for vitamin D deficiency in haemodialysis patients: effects on mineral metabolism and bone markers. *Nephrol Dial Transplant* Nov;23(11):3670–6. PMID: 18579534.

Jean, G., J. C. Terrat, T. Vanel, et al. 2008. Evidence for persistent vitamin D 1-alpha-hydroxylation in hemodialysis patients: evolution of serum 1,25-dihydroxycholecalciferol after 6 months of 25-hydroxycholecalciferol treatment. *Nephron Clin Pract* 110(1):c58–65. PMID: 18724068.

Frith, J. and J. L. Newton. 2009. Liver disease in older women. *Maturitas* Dec 2. [Epub ahead of print] PMID: 19962256.

99. Levey, A. S., L. A. Stevens, C. H. Schmid, et al. 2009. A new equation to estimate glomerular filtration rate. *Ann Intern Med* May 5;150(9):604–12. PMID: 19414839.

100. Frith, J., D. Jones and J. L. Newton. 2009. Chronic liver disease in an ageing population. *Age Ageing* Jan;38(1):11-8. Epub 2008 Nov 22. PMID: 19029099.

101. George, J., H. K. Ganesh, S. Acharya, et al. 2009. Bone mineral density and disorders of mineral metabolism in chronic liver disease. *World J Gastroenterol* Jul 28;15(28):3516–22. PMID: 19630107.

Murlikiewicz, K., A. Zawiasa, M. Nowicki. 2009. [Vitamin D—a panacea in nephrology and beyond] *Pol Merkur Lekarski* Nov;27(161):437–41. PMID: 19999813.

Moe, S. M., T. Drüeke, N. Lameire, et al. 2007. Chronic kidney disease-mineral-bone disorder: a new paradigm. *Adv Chronic Kidney Dis* Jan;14(1):3–12. PMID: 17200038.

Spasovski , G. B. 2007. Bone health and vascular calcification relationships in chronic kidney disease. *Int Urol Nephrol* 39(4):1209–16. Epub 2007 Sep 26. PMID: 17899431.

Jean, G., B. Charra and C. Chazot. 2008. Vitamin D deficiency and associated factors in hemodialysis patients. *J Ren Nutr* Sep;18(5):395–9. PMID: 18721733.

102. Braverman, E. R., T. J. Chen, A. L. Chen, et al. 2009. Age-related increases in parathyroid hormone may be antecedent to both osteoporosis and dementia. *BMC Endocr Disord* Oct 13;9:21. PMID: 19825157.

103. Bonjour, J. P., V. Benoit, O. Pourchaire, et al. 2009. Inhibition of markers of bone resorption by consumption of vitamin D and calcium-fortified soft plain cheese by institutionalised elderly women. *Br J Nutr* Oct;102(7):962–6. PMID: 19519975.

104. Braverman, E. R., T. J. Chen, A. L. Chen, et al. 2009. Age-related increases in parathyroid hormone may be antecedent to both osteoporosis and dementia. *BMC Endocr Disord* Oct 13;9:21. PMID: 19825157.

105. Williams, G. R. 2009. Actions of thyroid hormones in bone. *Endokrynol Pol* Sep-Oct;60(5):380–8. PMID: 19885809.

Zaidi, M., T. F. Davies, A. Zallone, H. C. Blair, et al. 2009. Thyroid-stimulating hormone, thyroid hormones, and bone loss. *Curr Osteoporos Rep* Jul;7(2):47–52. PMID: 19631028.

106. Suominen, H. 2006. Muscle training for bone strength. *Aging Clin Exp Res* Apr;18(2):85–93. PMID: 16702776.

107. Schmitt, N.M., J. Schmitt, M. Dören. 2009. The role of physical activity in the prevention of osteoporosis in postmenopausal women-An update. *Maturitas* May 20;63(1):34–8. Epub 2009 Apr 7. PMID: 19356867.

108. de Matos, O., D. J. Lopes da Silva, et al. 2009. Effect of specific exercise training on bone mineral density in women with postmenopausal osteopenia or osteoporosis. *Gynecol Endocrinol* Sep;25(9):616–20. PMID: 19533480.

109. Iwamoto, J., Y. Sato, T. Takeda, et al. 2009. Effectiveness of exercise in the treatment of lumbar spinal stenosis, knee osteoarthritis, and osteoporosis. *Aging Clin Exp Res* Nov 6. [Epub ahead of print] PMID: 19920410.

110. Brooke-Wavell. K., P. R. Jones, A. E. Hardman, et al. 2001. Commencing, continuing, and stopping brisk walking: effects on bone mineral density, quantitative ultrasound of bone and markers of bone metabolism in postmenopausal women. *Osteoporos Int* 12(7):581–7. PMID: 11527057.

111. Angin, E. and Z. Erden. 2009. [The effect of group exercise on postmenopausal osteoporosis and osteopenia] *Acta Orthop Traumatol Turc* Aug-Oct;43(4):343–50. PMID: 19809232.

112. Pizzorno, L. and J. Pizzorno. 2005. Clinical Pearls from the 12th Annual International Symposium on Functional Medicine, The Immune System Under Seige: New Clinical Approaches to Immunological Imbalances in the 21st Century, held May 26–28,

2005, Palm Springs, CA. Presentation by Michael Holick, How Vitamin D Modulates Immune and Inflammatory Processes. *IMCJ* Oct;4(5):30–33.

113. Guzel, R., E. Kozanoglu, F. Guler-Uysal, et al. 2001. Vitamin D status and bone mineral density of veiled and unveiled Turkish women. *J Womens Health Gend Based Med* Oct;10(8):765–70. PMID: 11703889.

Gannagé-Yared, M. H., G. Maalouf, S. Khalife, et al. 2009. Prevalence and predictors of vitamin D inadequacy amongst Lebanese osteoporotic women. *Br J Nutr* Feb;101(4):487–91.PMID: 18631414.

114. Binkley, N., R. Novotny, D. Krueger, et al. 2007. Low vitamin D status despite abundant sun exposure. *J Clin Endocrinol Metab* 92:2130–5. PMID: 17426097.

115. Gannagé-Yared, M. H., G. Maalouf, S. Khalife, et al. 2009. Prevalence and predictors of vitamin D inadequacy amongst Lebanese osteoporotic women. *Br J Nutr* Feb;101(4):487–91.PMID: 18631414.

116. Chapuy, M. C., M. E. Arlot, P. D. Delmas, et al. 1994. Effect of calcium and cholecalciferol treatment for three years on hip fractures in elderly women. *BMJ* Apr 23;308(6936):1081–2. PMID: 8173430.

117. Chapuy, M. C., M. E. Arlot, F. Duboeuf , et al. 1992. Vitamin D3 and calcium to prevent hip fractures in the elderly women. *N Engl J Med* Dec 3;327(23):1637–42. PMID: 1331788.

Meunier, P. J., M. C. Chapuy, M. E. Arlot, et al. 1994. Can we stop bone loss and prevent hip fractures in the elderly? *Osteoporos Int* 4 Suppl 1:71–6. PMID: 8081065.

118. Chapuy, M. C., R. Pamphile, E. Paris, et al. 2002. Combined calcium and vitamin D3 supplementation in elderly women: confirmation of reversal of secondary hyperparathyroidism and hip fracture risk: the Decalyos II study. *Osteoporos Int* Mar;13(3):257–64. PMID: 11991447.

119. http://www.vitamindcouncil.org.

120. Legroux-Gérot, I., J. Vignau, M. D'Herbomez, et al. 2007. Evaluation of bone loss and its mechanisms in anorexia nervosa. *Calcif Tissue Int* Sep;81(3):174–82. PMID: 17668143.

Legroux-Gérot, I., J. Vignau, E. Biver, et al. 2010. Anorexia nervosa, osteoporosis and circulating leptin: the missing link. *Osteoporos Int* Jan 6. [Epub ahead of print] PMID: 20052458.

121. Loke, Y. K., S. Singh, C. D. Furberg. 2009. Long-term use of thiazolidinediones and fractures in type 2 diabetes: a meta-analysis. *CMAJ* Jan 6;180(1):32–9. PMID: 19073651.

Dormuth, C. R., G. Carney, B. Carleton, et al. 2009. Thiazolidinediones and fractures in men and women. *Arch Intern Med* Aug 10;169(15):1395–402. PMID: 19667303.

Douglas, I. J., S. J. Evans, S. Pocock, et al. 2009. The risk of fractures associated with thiazolidinediones: a self-controlled case-series study. *PLoS Med* Sep;6(9):e1000154. PMID: 19787025.

Meier, C., M. Bodmer, C. R. Meier, et al. 2009. [Thiazolidinediones and skeletal health] *Rev Med Suisse* Jun 10;5(207):1309–10, 1312–3. PMID: 19626930.

122. McDonough, A. K., R. S. Rosenthal, et al. 2008. The effect of thiazolidinediones on BMD and osteoporosis. *Nat Clin Pract Endocrinol Metab* Sep;4(9):507–13. PMID: 18695700.

123. Daniell, H. W. 2008. Opioid endocrinopathy in women consuming prescribed sustained-action opioids for control of nonmalignant pain. *J Pain* Jan;9(1):28–36. PMID: 17936076.

Vuong, C., S. H. Van Uum, L. E. O'Dell, et al. 2010. The effects of opioids and opioid analogs on animal and human endocrine systems. *Endocr Rev* Feb;31(1):98–132. PMID: 19903933.

Katz, N., N. A. Mazer. 2009. The impact of opioids on the endocrine system. *Clin J Pain* Feb;25(2):170–5. PMID: 19333165.

Bassett, J. H., P. J. O'Shea, S. Sriskantharajah, et al. 2007. Thyroid hormone excess rather than thyrotropin deficiency induces osteoporosis in hyperthyroidism. *Mol Endocrinol* May;21(5):1095–107. PMID: 17327419.

Zaidi, M., T. F. Davies, A. Zallone, et al. 2009. Thyroid-stimulating hormone, thyroid hormones, and bone loss. *Curr Osteoporos Rep* Jul;7(2):47–52. PMID: 19631028.

124. Weng, M.Y., N. E. Lane. 2007. Medication-induced osteoporosis. *Curr Osteoporos Rep* Dec;5(4):139–45. PMID: 18430387.

De Nijs, R. N. 2008. Glucocorticoid-induced osteoporosis: a review on pathophysiology and treatment options. *Minerva Med* Feb;99(1):23–43. PMID: 18299694.

Silverman, S.L., N. E. Lane. 2009. Glucocorticoid-induced osteoporosis. *Curr Osteoporos Rep* Mar;7(1):23–6. PMID: 19239826.

125. Slemenda, C.W., S. L. Hui, C. Longcope and C. C. Johnston, Jr. 1989. Cigarette smoking, obesity, and bone mass. *J Bone Miner Res* Oct;4(5):737–41. PMID: 2816518.

Krall, E. A. and B. Dawson-Hughes. 1991. Smoking and bone loss among postmenopausal women. *J Bone Miner Res* Apr;6(4):331–8. PMID: 1858519.

Vestergaard, P. and L. Mosekilde. 2003. Fracture risk associated with smoking: a meta-analysis. *J Intern Med* Dec;254(6):572–83. PMID: 14641798.

Ward, K. D. and R. C. Klesges. 2001. A meta-analysis of the effects of cigarette smoking on bone mineral density. *Calcif Tissue Int* May;68(5):259–70. PMID: 11683532.

126. Høidrup, S., E. Prescott, T. I. Sørensen, et al. 2000. Tobacco smoking and risk of hip fracture in men and women. *Int J Epidemiol* Apr;29(2):253–9. PMID: 10817121.

127. Seeman, E., L. J. Melton, 3rd, W. M. O'Fallon, et al. 1983. Risk factors for spinal osteoporosis in men. *Am J Med* Dec;75(6):977–83. PMID: 6650552.

128. Kazantzis, G. 2004. Cadmium, osteoporosis, and calcium metabolism. *Biometals* Oct;17(5):493–8. PMID: 15688852.

129. Friberg, L. 1983. Cadmium. *Annu Rev Public Health* 4:367–73. PMID: 6860444.

130. Apeti, D. A., G. G. Lauenstein and G. F. Riedel. 2009. Cadmium distribution in coastal sediments and mollusks of the US. *Mar Pollut Bull* Jul;58(7):1016–24. PMID: 19342067.

131. Wilkinson, J. M., J. Hill and C. J. Phillips. 2003. The accumulation of potentially toxic metals by grazing ruminants. *Proc Nutr Soc* May;62(2):267–77. PMID: 14506874.

132. Akesson, A., P. Bjellerup, T. Lundh, et al. 2006. Cadmium-induced effects on bone in a population-based study of women. *Environ Health Perspect* Jun;114(6):830–4. PMID: 16759980.

McElroy, J. A., M. M. Shafer, J. M. Hampton, et al. 2007. Predictors of urinary cadmium levels in adult females. *Sci Total Environ* Sep 1;382(2–3):214–23. PMID: 17544058.

133. Hogervorst, J., M. Plusquin, J. Vangronsveld, et al. 2007. House dust as possible route of environmental exposure to cadmium and lead in the adult general population. *Environ Res* Jan;103(1):30–7. PMID: 16843453.

134. "US Agency Goes After Cadmium in Children's Jewelry," http://abcnews.go.com/Health/ WellnessNews/wireStory?id=9527916 (accessed 3-2-10).

"Cadmium: The New Made-in-China Scare," http://www.businessweek.com/globalbiz/blog/ eyeonasia/archives/2010/01/cadmium_the_ new.html.

"U.S. to Develop Safety Standards for Toxic Metals," (Update 2), http://www.businessweek.com/ news/2010-01-12/u-s-to-develop-safety-standards-for-toxic-metals-update1-.html.

135. Andujar, P., L. Bensefa-Colas, A. Descatha. 2009. [Acute and chronic cadmium poisoning.] *Rev Med Interne* Aug 24. [Epub ahead of print] PMID: 19709784.

Järup, L., A. Akesson. 2009. Current status of cadmium as an environmental health problem. *Toxicol Appl Pharmacol* Aug 1;238(3):201–8. Epub 2009 May 3. PMID: 19409405.

136. Gallagher, C. M., J. S. Kovach, J. R. Meliker. 2008. Urinary cadmium and osteoporosis in U.S. Women >or= 50 years of age: NHANES 1988– 1994 and 1999–2004. *Environ Health Perspect* Oct;116(10):1338–43. PMID: 18941575.

137. Laroche, M., Y. Lasne, A. Felez, L. Moulinier, et al. 1994. [Osteocalcin and smoking] *Rev Rhum Ed Fr* Jun;61(6):433–6. PMID: 7833868.

138. Lee, N. K., H. Sowa, E. Hinoi, et al. 2007. Endocrine regulation of energy metabolism by the

skeleton. *Cell* Aug 10;130(3):456–69. PMID: 17693256.

Wolf, G. 2008. Energy regulation by the skeleton. *Nutr Rev* Apr;66(4):229–33. PMID: 18366536.

139. Rothem, D. E., L. Rothem, M. Soudry, et al. 2009. Nicotine modulates bone metabolism-associated gene expression in osteoblast cells. *J Bone Miner Metab* 27(5):555–61. PMID: 19436947.

Kamer, A. R., N. El-Ghorab, N. Marzec, et al. 2006. Nicotine induced proliferation and cytokine release in osteoblastic cells. *Int J Mol Med* Jan;17(1):121–7. PMID: 16328020.

140. Mueck, A. O., H. Seeger. 2005. Smoking, estradiol metabolism, and hormone replacement therapy. *Curr Med Chem Cardiovasc Hematol Agents* Jan;3(1):45–54. PMID: 15638743.

141. Benson, B. W. and J. D. Shulman. 2005. Inclusion of tobacco exposure as a predictive factor for decreased bone mineral content. *Nicotine Tob Res* Oct;7(5):719–24. PMID: 16191742.

142. Oncken, C., K. Prestwood, A. Kleppinger, et al. 2006. Impact of smoking cessation on bone mineral density in postmenopausal women. *J Womens Health* (Larchmt) Dec;15(10):1141–50. PMID: 17199455.

143. Chakkalakal, D. A. 2005. Alcohol-induced bone loss and deficient bone repair. *Alcohol Clin Exp Res* Dec;29(12):2077–90. PMID: 16385177.

Broulik, P. D., J. Rosenkrancová, P. Růžička, et al. 2009. The effect of chronic alcohol administration on bone mineral content and bone strength in male rats. *Physiol Res* Nov 20. [Epub ahead of print] PMID: 19929136.

144. Wosje, K. S. and H. J. Kalkwarf. 2007. Bone density in relation to alcohol intake among men and women in the United States. *Osteoporos Int* Mar;18(3):391–400. PMID: 17091218.

145. Kanis, J. A., H. Johansson, O. Johnell, et al. 2005. Alcohol intake as a risk factor for fracture. *Osteoporos Int* Jul;16(7):737–42. PMID: 15455194.

146. Pedrera-Zamorano, J. D., J. M. Lavado-Garcia, R. Roncero-Martin, et al. 2009. Effect of beer drinking on ultrasound bone mass in women. *Nutrition* Oct;25(10):1057–63. Epub 2009 Jun 13. PMID: 19527924.

147. Tucker, K. L., 2009. Jugdaohsingh R, Powell JJ, et al. Effects of beer, wine, and liquor intakes on bone mineral density in older men and women. *Am J Clin Nutr* Apr;89(4):1188–96. Epub 2009 Feb 25. PMID: 19244365.

Liu, Z. P., W. X. Li, B. Yu, et al. 2005. Effects of trans-resveratrol from Polygonum cuspidatum on bone loss using the ovariectomized rat model. *J Med Food Spring* 8(1):14-9. PMID: 15857203.

King, R. E., J. A. Bomser and D. B. Min. Bioactivity of resveratrol. Compr Rev Food Sci Food Saf 5:65–70. DOI 10.1111/j.1541-4337.2006.00001.x , http://www3.interscience.wiley.com/journal/118607162/abstract.

148. Binkley, N. 2009. A perspective on male osteoporosis. *Best Pract Res Clin Rheumatol* Dec;23(6):755–68. PMID: 19945687.

149. Binkley, N. 2006. Osteoporosis in men. *Arq Bras Endocrinol Metabol* Aug;50(4):764–74. PMID: 17117301.

150. Orwoll, E., C. M. Nielson, L. M. Marshall, et al. 2009. Vitamin D deficiency in older men. *J Clin Endocrinol Metab* Apr;94(4):1214–22. PMID: 19174492.

151. van Hogezand, R. A., N. A. Hamdy. 2006. Skeletal morbidity in inflammatory bowel disease. *Scand J Gastroenterol Suppl* May;(243):59–64. PMID: 16782623.

152. Orlic, Z. C., T. Turk, B. M. Sincic, et al. 2010. How activity of inflammatory bowel disease influences bone loss. *J Clin Densitom* Jan-Mar;13(1):36–42. PMID: 20171567.

153. Liu, G., M. Peacock, O. Eilam, et al. 1997. Effect of osteoarthritis in the lumbar spine and hip on bone mineral density and diagnosis of osteoporosis in elderly men and women. *Osteoporos Int* 7(6):564–9. PMID: 9604053.

154. Khosla, S., S. Amin, E. Orwoll. 2008. Osteoporosis in men. *Endocr Rev* Jun;29(4):441–64. PMID: 18451258 Clarke BL, Khosla S. Androgens and bone. *Steroids.* 2009 Mar;74(3):296–305. PMID: 18992761.

155. Binkley, N. 2006. Osteoporosis in men. *Arq Bras Endocrinol Metabol* Aug;50(4):764–74. PMID: 17117301.

156. Shahinian, V. B., Y. F. Kuo, J. L. Freeman, et al. 2005. Risk of fracture after androgen deprivation for prostate cancer. *N Engl J Med* Jan 13;352(2):154–64. PMID: 15647578.

157. *Assessment of Fracture Risk and Its Application to Screening for Postmenopausal Osteoporosis.* (Geneva: WHO,1994).

158. Ahuja, J., D. Rhodes, D. Goldman, et al. Intakes and sources of vitamin D in the US population. http://www.fasebj.org/cgi/content/meeting_abstract/24/1_MeetingAbstracts/917.6?maxtoshow=&hits=20&RESULTFORMAT=&searchid=1&FIRSTINDEX=0&displaysectionid=Calcium%2C+Phosphorus%2C+Magnesium%2C+and+Vitamin+D&volume=24&issue=1_MeetingAbstracts&resourcetype=HWCIT (accessed 5-11-2010).

159. Bischoff-Ferrari, H. A. 2008. Optimal serum 25-hydroxyvitamin D levels for multiple health outcomes. *Adv Exp Med Biol* 624:55–71. PMID: 18348447.

160. Mistretta, V. I., P. Delanaye, J. P. Chapelle JP, et al. 2008. [Vitamin D2 or vitamin D3?] *Rev Med Interne* Oct;29(10):815–20. PMID: 18406498.

161. Vieth, R. 2007. Vitamin D toxicity, policy, and science. *J Bone Miner Res* Dec;22 Suppl 2:V64–8. PMID: 18290725.

162. Mundy, G. R. 2007. Osteoporosis and inflammation. *Nutr Rev* Dec;65(12 Pt 2):S147–51. PMID: 18240539.

Shea, M. K., S. L. Booth, J. M. Massaro, et al. 2008. Vitamin K and vitamin D status: associations with inflammatory markers in the Framingham Offspring Study. *Am J Epidemiol* Feb 1;167(3):313–20. PMID: 18006902.

163. Pizzorno, L. Vitamin K, *Longevity Medicine Review*, 2009, http://www.lmreview.com/articles/view/vitamin-k/.

Pizzorno, L. Vitamin K2, but not vitamin K1, is helpful for bone density. *Longevity Medicine Review* 2009, http://www.lmreview.com/articles/view/vitamin-k2-but-not-vitamin-k1-is-helpful-for-bone-density/.

Pizzorno, L. Vitamin D and Vitamin K team up to lower CVD risk: Part I, *Longevity Medicine Review* 2009, http://www.lmreview.com/articles/view/vitamin-d-and-vitamin-k-team-up-to-lower-cvd-risk-part-1/.

Pizzorno, L. Vitamin D and Vitamin K team up to lower CVD risk: Part 2, *Longevity Medicine Review* 2009, http://www.lmreview.com/articles/view/vitamin-d-and-vitamin-k-team-up-to-lower-cvd-risk-part-2/.

164. Hart, J. P., A. Catterall, R. A. Dodds, et al. 1984. Circulating vitamin K1 levels in fractured neck of femur. *Lancet* Aug 4;2(8397):283. PMID: 6146829.

Hodges, S. J., M. J. Pilkington, T. C. Stamp, et al. 1991. Depressed levels of circulating menaquinones in patients with osteoporotic fractures of the spine and femoral neck. *Bone* 12(6):387–9. PMID: 1797053.

165. Booth, S. L., K. L. Tucker, H. Chen, et al. 2000. Dietary vitamin K intakes are associated with hip fracture but not with bone mineral density in elderly men and women. *Am J Clin Nutr* May;71(5):1201–8. PMID: 10799384.

166. Iinuma, N. 2005. [Vitamin K2 (menatetrenone) and bone quality] *Clin Calcium* Jun;15(6):1034–9. PMID: 15930719.

167. Plaza, S. M., D. W. Lamson. 2005. Vitamin K2 in bone metabolism and osteoporosis. *Altern Med Rev* Mar;10(1):24–35. PMID: 15771560.

168. Cockayne, S., J. Adamson, S. Lanham-New, et al. 2006. Vitamin K and the prevention of fractures: systematic review and meta-analysis of randomized controlled trials. *Arch Intern Med* Jun 26;166(12):1256–61. PMID: 16801507.

169. Pizzorno, L. 2008. Vitamin K: beyond coagulation to uses in bone, vascular and anti-cancer metabolism, *IMCJ* Apr; 7(2): 24–30.

170. Iwamoto, J., T. Takeda and S. Ichimura. 2000. Effect of combined administration of vitamin D3 and vitamin K2 on bone mineral density of the lumbar spine in postmenopausal women with osteoporosis. *J Orthop Sci* 5(6):546–51. PMID: 11180916.

171. Ushiroyama, T., A. Ikeda and M. Ueki. 2002. Effect of continuous combined therapy with vitamin K(2) and vitamin D(3) on bone mineral density and coagulofibrinolysis function in post-

menopausal women. *Maturitas* Mar 25;41(3): 211–21. PMID: 11886767.

172. McCann, J. C. and B. N. Ames. 2009. Vitamin K, an example of triage theory: is micronutrient inadequacy linked to diseases of aging? *Am J Clin Nutr* Oct;90(4):889–907. PMID: 19692494.

173. Source: Food Processor Version 7.60, *ESHA Research*, Salem, OR, December 2000.

174. Pizzorno, L. 2008. Vitamin K: beyond coagulation to uses in bone, vascular and anti-cancer metabolism, *IMCJ* Apr; 7(2): 24–30.

175. Natto, http://en.wikipedia.org/wiki/Natt%C5%8D (accessed 5-13-10).

176. Forli, L., J. Bollerslev, S. Simonsen, et al. 2010. Dietary vitamin K2 supplement improves bone status after lung and heart transplantation. *Transplantation.* 2010 Feb 27;89(4):458–64. PMID: 20177349.

177. Yamaguchi, M. 2006. Regulatory mechanism of food factors in bone metabolism and prevention of osteoporosis. *Yakugaku Zasshi.* 2006 Nov; 126(11): 1117–37. PMID: 17077614.

178. Food and Nutrition Board, Institute of Medicine. Vitamin K. Dietary Reference Intakes for Vitamin A, Vitamin K, Arsenic, Boron, Chromium, Copper, Iodine, Iron, Manganese, Molybdenum, Nickel, Silicon, Vanadium, and Zinc. Washington, D.C. *National Academy Press* 2001:162–196, http://www.nap.edu/openbook. php?isbn=0309072794.

179. Schurgers, L. J., K. J. Teunissen and K. Hamulyák. 2007. Vitamin K-containing dietary supplements: comparison of synthetic vitamin K1 and natto-derived menaquinone-7. *Blood Apr* 15;109(8):3279–83. PMID: 17158229.

Schurgers, L. J. Vitamin K2 as MenaQ7, Improve bone health and inhibit arterial calcification. Monograph published April 2007, *NattoPharma*, ASA, Norway, http://www.menaq7.com/index. php?s=Research.

180. IOM Report: Dietary Reference Intakes for Vitamin A, Vitamin K, Arsenic, Boron, Chromium, Copper, Iodine, Iron, Manganese, Molybdenum, Nickel, Silicon, Vanadium, and Zinc, http:// www.iom.edu/~/media/Files/Activity%20Files/ Nutrition/DRIs/DRI_Vitamins.ashx.

181. McCormick, R. K. 2007. Osteoporosis: integrating biomarkers and other diagnostic correlates into the management of bone fragility. *Altern Med Rev* Jun;12(2):113–45. PMID: 17604458.

182. Koh, J. M., Y. S. Lee, Y. S. Kim, et al. 2006. Homocysteine enhances bone resorption by stimulation of osteoclast formation and activity through increased intracellular ROS generation. *J Bone Miner Res* Jul;21(7):1003–11. PMID: 16813521.

Kim, D. J., J. M. Koh, O. Lee, et al. 2006. Homocysteine enhances apoptosis in human bone marrow stromal cells. *Bone* Sep 39(3):582–90. PMID: 16644300.

183. Lee, N. K., Y. G. Choi, J. Y. Baik, et al. 2005. A crucial role for reactive oxygen species in RANKL-induced osteoclast differentiation, *Blood* 106, pp. 852–859. PMID: 15817678.

Ginaldi, L., M. C. Di Benedetto, M. De Martinis. 2005. Osteoporosis, inflammation and ageing. *Immun Ageing* 2:14. PMID: 16271143.

184. Choi, K. M., Y. K. Seo, H. H. Yoon, et al. 2008. Effect of ascorbic acid on bone marrow-derived mesenchymal stem cell proliferation and differentiation. *J Biosci Bioeng* Jun;105(6):586–94. PMID: 18640597.

Sahni, S., M. T. Hannan, D. Gagnon, et al. 2008. High vitamin C intake is associated with lower 4-year bone loss in elderly men. *J Nutr* Oct;138(10):1931–8. PMID: 18806103.

185. Ibid.

186. Rowe, D. J., S. Ko, X. M. Tom, et al. 1999. Enhanced production of mineralized nodules and collagenous proteins in vitro by calcium ascorbate supplemented with vitamin C metabolites. *J Periodontol* Sep;70(9):992–9. PMID: 10505801.

187. Prevalence and Incidence of Iron deficiency anemia, http://www.wrongdiagnosis.com/i/iron_deficiency_anemia/prevalence.htm#incidence_intro (accessed 5-13-10).

188. National Osteoporosis Foundation, What You Should Know About Calcium, http://www.nof.org/prevention/calcium2.htm (accessed 5-13-10).

189. Pizorno, J. E. and M. T. Murray., "Osteoporosis," in the *Textbook of Natural Medicine*, 3rd ed.,: (St Louis, MO: Churchill Livingstone, 2006), chap 146.

National Institutes of Health. 2000. Osteoporosis prevention, diagnosis, and therapy. *NIH Consensus Statement* Mar 27–29;17(1):1–45.

Xu, L., P. McElduff, C. D'Este and J. Attia. 2004. Does dietary calcium have a protective effect on bone fractures in women? A meta-analysis of observational studies. *Br J Nutr* 91:625–634. PMID: 15035690.

Reid, I. R., R. W. Ames, M. C. Evans, et al. 1995. Long-term effects of calcium supplementation on bone loss and fractures in postmenopausal women: a randomized controlled trial. *Am J Med* 98:331–335. PMID: 7709944.

Devine, A., I. M. Dick, S. J. Heal, et al. 1997. A 4-year follow-up study of the effects of calcium supplementation on bone density in elderly postmenopausal women. *Osteoporos Int* 7:23–28. PMID: 9102058.

Elders, P. J., P. Lips, J. C. Netelenbos, et al. 1994. Long-term effect of calcium supplementation on bone loss in perimenopausal women. *J Bone Miner Res* 9:963–970. PMID: 7942164.

190. Shea, B., G. Wells, A. Cranney, et al. 2007. WITHDRAWN: Calcium supplementation on bone loss in postmenopausal women. *Cochrane Database Syst Rev* Jul 18;(1):CD004526. PMID: 17636765.

191. Bourgoin, B. P., D. R. Evans, J. R. Cornett, et al. 1993. Lead content in 70 brands of dietary calcium supplements. *Am J Public Health* 83:1155–1160. PMID: 8342726.

Scelfo, G. M. and A. R. Flegal. 2000. Lead in calcium supplements. *Environ Health Perspect* Apr;108(4):309–19. PMID: 10753088.

192. Pizzorno, L. U., J. E. Pizzorno and M. T. Murray. "Osteoporosis", in *Natural Medicine Instructions for Patients*, (Churchill Livingstone/Elsevier, 2002), p. 251–9.

193. Pounder, R. E. and D. Ng. The prevalence of Helicobacter pylori infection in different countries. *Aliment Pharmacol Ther* 9 Suppl 2:33–9. PMID: 8547526.

194. Straub, D. A. 2007. Calcium supplementation in clinical practice: a review of forms, doses, and indications. *Nutr Clin Pract* Jun;22(3):286–96. PMID: 17507729.

195. World's Healthiest Foods, Calcium, http://www.whfoods.org/genpage.php?tname=nutrient&dbid=45 (accessed 5-16-2010).

Linus Pauling Institute, Calcium, http://lpi.oregonstate.edu/infocenter/minerals/calcium/ (accessed 5-16-2010).

196. Castelo-Branco, C., M. Ciria-Recasens, M. J. Cancelo-Hidalgo, et al. 2009. Efficacy of ossein-hydroxyapatite complex compared with calcium carbonate to prevent bone loss: a meta-analysis. *Menopause* Sep-Oct;16(5):984–91. PMID: 19407667

197. Pines, A., H. Raafat, A. H. Lynn and J.Whittington J. 1984. Clinical trial of microcrystalline hydroxy-apatite compound ('Ossopan') in the prevention of osteoporosis due to corticosteroid therapy. *Curr Med Res Opin* 8(10):734–42. PMID: 6373153.

Stellon, A., A. Davies, A. Webb and R. Williams. 1985. Microcrystalline hydroxyapatite compound in prevention of bone loss in corticosteroid-treated patients with chronic active hepatitis. *Postgrad Med J* Sep;61(719):791–6. PMID: 2997764.

198. Nielsen, F. H., B. J. Stoecker. 2009. *J Trace Elem Med Biol* 23(3):195–203. PMID: 19486829; And Nielsen F.H. 2008. Is boron nutritionally relevant? *Nutr Rev* Apr;66(4):183–91. PMID: 18366532.

Gorustovich, A. A., T. Steimetz, F. H. Nielsen, et al. 2008. Histomorphometric study of alveolar bone healing in rats fed a boron-deficient diet. *Anat Rec* (Hoboken) Apr;291(4):441–7. PMID: 18361451.

Nielsen, F. H. 2000. The emergence of boron as nutritionally important throughout the life cycle. *Nutrition* Jul-Aug;16(7–8):512–4. PMID: 10906539.

Nielsen, F. H. 2009. Micronutrients in parenteral nutrition: boron, silicon, and fluoride. *Gastroenterology* Nov;137(5 Suppl):S55–60. PMID: 19874950.

Nielsen, F. H. and B. J. Stoecker. 2009. Boron and fish oil have different beneficial effects on strength and trabecular microarchitecture of bone. *J Trace Elem Med Biol* 23(3):195–203. PMID: 19486829.

199. Samman, S., M. R. Naghii, Lyons Wall PM, et al. 1998. The nutritional and metabolic effects of boron in humans and animals. *Biol Trace Elem Res* Winter;66(1–3):227–35. PMID: 10050922.

Schaafsma, A., P. J. de Vries and W. H. Saris. 2001. Delay of natural bone loss by higher intakes of specific minerals and vitamins. *Crit Rev Food Sci Nutr* May;41(4):225–49. PMID: 11401244.

Nielsen, F. H. 1990. Studies on the relationship between boron and magnesium which possibly affects the formation and maintenance of bones. *Magnes Trace Elem* 9(2):61–9. PMID: 2222801.

200. Nielsen, F. H., C. D. Hunt, L. M. Mullen, et al. 1987. Effect of dietary boron on mineral, estrogen, and testosterone metabolism in postmenopausal women. *FASEB J* Nov;1(5):394–7. PMID: 3678698.

201. Dietary Reference Intakes for Vitamin A, Vitamin K, Arsenic, Boron, Chromium, Copper, Iodine, Iron, Manganese, Molybdenum, Nickel, Silicon, Vanadium, and Zinc. 2001. *Food and Nutrition Board, Institute of Medicine*, available at http://books.nap.edu/openbook.php?record_id=10026&page=1 (accessed 5-13-10).

202. Johnson, S. 2001. The multifaceted and wide-spread pathology of magnesium deficiency. *Med Hypotheses* Feb;56(2):163–70. PMID: 11425281.

203. Rude, R. K., F. R. Singer and H. E. Gruber. 2009. Skeletal and hormonal effects of magnesium deficiency. *J Am Coll Nutr* Apr;28(2):131–41. PMID: 19828898.

204. Rude, R. K., J. S. Adams, E. Ryzen, et al. 1985. Low serum concentrations of 1,25-dihydroxyvitamin D in human magnesium deficiency. *J Clin Endocrinol Metab* Nov;61(5):933–40. PMID: 3840173.

205. Rude, R. K., F. R. Singer and H. E. Gruber. 2009. Skeletal and hormonal effects of magnesium deficiency. *J Am Coll Nutr* Apr;28(2):131–41. PMID: 19828898.

206. World's Healthiest Foods, Magnisium, http://www.whfoods.org/genpage.php?tname=nutrient&dbid=75 (accessed 5-16-2010).

   Magnesium, Eat Right Ontario, https://www.eat-rightontario.ca/en/viewdocument.aspx?id=67 (accessed 5-16-2010).

207. Cohen, L. and R. Kitzes. 1981. Infrared spectroscopy and magnesium content of bone mineral in osteoporotic women. Infrared spectroscopy and magnesium content of bone mineral in osteoporotic women. *Isr J Med Sci* Dec;17(12):1123–5. PMID: 7327911.

   Cohen, L. 1988. Recent data on magnesium and osteoporosis. *Magnes Res* Jul;1(1–2):85–7. PMID: 3079205.

Launius, B.K., P. A. Brown, E. M. Cush, et al. 2004. Osteoporosis: The dynamic relationship between magnesium and bone mineral density in the heart transplant patient. *Crit Care Nurs Q* Jan-Mar;27(1):96–100. PMID: 14974529.

Takami, M. and S. Shinnichi. 2005. [Bone and magnesium] *Clin Calcium* Nov;15(11):91–6. PMID: 16272618.

208. Musayev, F.N., M. L. Di Salvo, M. A. Saavedra, et al. 2009. Molecular basis of reduced pyridoxine 5'-phosphate oxidase catalytic activity in neonatal epileptic encephalopathy disorder. *J Biol Chem* Nov 6;284(45):30949–56. PMID: 19759001.

Khayat, M., S. H. Korman, P. Frankel, et al. 2008. PNPO deficiency: an under diagnosed inborn error of pyridoxine metabolism. *Mol Genet Metab* Aug;94(4):431–4. PMID: 18485777.

Hoey, L., H. McNulty and J. J. Strain. 2009. Studies of biomarker responses to intervention with riboflavin: a systematic review. *Am J Clin Nutr* Jun;89(6):1960S-1980S. PMID: 19403631.

209. Reginster, J. Y., R. Deroisy, M. Dougados, et al. 2002. Prevention of early postmenopausal bone loss by strontium ranelate: the randomized, two-year, double-masked, dose-ranging, placebo-controlled PREVOS trial. *Osteoporos Int* Dec;13(12):925–31. PMID: 12459934.

210. Seeman, E., J. Devogelaer, R. Lorenc, et al. 2008. Strontium ranelate reduces the risk of vertebral

fractures in patients with osteopenia. *J Bone Miner Res* Mar;23(3):433–8. PMID: 17997711.

211. Meunier, P., C. Roux, S. Ortolani, et al. 2009. Effects of long-term strontium ranelate treatment on vertebral fracture risk in postmenopausal women with osteoporosis. *Osteoporos Int* Oct;20(10):1663–73. PMID: 19153678.

Meunier, P., C. Roux, E. Seeman, et al. 2004. The effects of strontium ranelate on the risk of vertebral fracture in women with postmenopausal osteoporosis. *N Engl J Med* Jan 29;350(5):459–68. PMID: 14749454.

Reginster, J., E. Seeman, M. C. De Vernejoul, et al. 2005. Strontium ranelate reduces the risk of nonvertebral fractures in postmenopausal women with osteoporosis: Treatment of Peripheral Osteoporosis (TROPOS) study. *J Clin Endocrinol Metab* May;90(5):2816–22. Epub 2005 Feb 22. PMID: 15728210.

212. Arlot, M. E., Y. Jiang, H. K. Genant, et al. 2008. Histomorphometric and microCT analysis of bone biopsies from postmenopausal osteoporotic women treated with strontium ranelate. *J Bone Miner Res* Feb;23(2):215–22. PMID: 17922612.

213. Seeman, E., J. Devogelaer, R. Lorenc, et al. 2008. Strontium ranelate reduces the risk of vertebral fractures in patients with osteopenia. *J Bone Miner Res* Mar;23(3):433–8. PMID: 17997711.

214. Neuprez, A., J. Y. Reginster. 2008. Bone-forming agents in the management of osteoporosis. *Best*

Pract Res Clin Endocrinol Metab Oct;22(5):869–83. PMID: 19028361.

215. Liu, J. M., A. Wai-Chee Kung, et al. 2009. Efficacy and safety of 2 g/day of strontium ranelate in Asian women with postmenopausal osteoporosis. *Bone* Sep;45(3):460–5. Epub 2009 May 21. PMID: 19464401.

216. Middleton, E. T., S. A. Steel, M. Aye, et al. 2010. The effect of prior bisphosphonate therapy on the subsequent BMD and bone turnover response to strontium ranelate. *J Bone Miner Res* Mar;25(3):455–62. PMID: 20201000.

217. Patnaik, P. *Handbook of Inorganic Chemicals* (McGraw-Hill, 2002), ISBN 0070494398.

218. Marie, P. J. 2006. Strontium ranelate: a dual mode of action rebalancing bone turnover in favour of bone formation. *Curr Opin Rheumatol* Jun;18 Suppl 1:S11–5. PMID: 16735840.

Marie, P. J. 2006. Strontium ranelate: a physiological approach for optimizing bone formation and resorption. *Bone* Feb;38(2 Suppl 1):S10–4. Epub 2006 Jan 24. PMID: 16439191.

Boivin, G. and P. J. Meunier. 2003. The mineralization of bone tissue: a forgotten dimension in osteoporosis research. *Osteoporos Int* 14 Suppl 3:S19–24. Epub 2003 Mar 18. Review. PMID: 12730799.

Boivin, G., D. Farlay, M. T. Khebbab, et al. 2010. In osteoporotic women treated with strontium ranelate, strontium is located in bone formed during treatment with a maintained degree of mineralization. *Osteoporos Int.* Apr;21(4):667–77. Epub 2009 Jul 14. PMID: 19597910.

Uebelhart, D., D. Frey, P. Frey-Rindova, et al. 2003. [Therapy of osteoporosis: bisphosphonates, SERM's, teriparatide and strontium] *Z Rheumatol* Dec;62(6):512–7. PMID: 14685711.

219. Deeks, E. D., S. Dhillon. 2010. Strontium ranelate: a review of its use in the treatment of postmenopausal osteoporosis. *Drugs* Apr 16;70(6):733–59. PMID: 20394457.

220. Musette, P., M. L. Brandi, P. Cacoub, et al. 2010. Treatment of osteoporosis: recognizing and managing cutaneous adverse reactions and drug-induced hypersensitivity. *Osteoporos Int* May;21(5):723–32. Epub 2009 Nov 17. PMID: 19921087.

Pernicova, I., E. T. Middleton and M. Aye. 2008. Rash, strontium ranelate and DRESS syndrome put into perspective. European Medicine Agency on the alert. *Osteoporos Int* Dec;19(12):1811–2. Epub 2008 Sep 20. PMID: 18807101.

Kramkimel, N., C. Sibon, C. Le Beller, et al. 2009. *Clin Exp Dermatol* Oct;34(7):e349–50. Epub 2009 May 16. PMID: 19456761.

Jonville-Béra, A. P., B. Crickx, L. Aaron, et al. 2009. Strontium ranelate-induced DRESS syndrome: first two case reports. *Allergy* Apr;64(4):658–9. Epub 2009 Feb 7. PMID: 19210353.

Iyer, D., Y. Buggy, K. O'Reilly, et al. 2009. Strontium ranelate as a cause of acute renal failure and dress syndrome. *Nephrology* (Carlton) Sep;14(6):624. PMID: 19712264.

221. Chen, F. P., K. C. Wang and J. D. Huang. 2009. Effect of estrogen on the activity and growth of human osteoclasts in vitro. Taiwan *J Obstet Gynecol* Dec;48(4):350–5. PMID: 20045755.

Imai, Y., M. Y. Youn, S. Kondoh, et al. 2009. Estrogens maintain bone mass by regulating expression of genes controlling function and life span in mature osteoclasts. *Ann N Y Acad Sci* Sep;1173 Suppl 1:E31–9. PMID: 19751412.

McLean, R. R. 2009. Proinflammatory cytokines and osteoporosis. *Curr Osteoporos Rep* Dec;7(4):134–9. PMID: 19968917.

Boyce, B. F. and L. Xing. 2008. Functions of RANKL/RANK/OPG in bone modeling and remodeling. *Arch Biochem Biophys* May 15;473(2):139–46. Epub 2008 Mar 25. PMID: 18395508.

Mundy, G. R. 2007. Osteoporosis and inflammation. *Nutr Rev* Dec;65(12 Pt 2):S147–51. PMID: 18240539.

D'Amelio, P., A. Grimaldi, S. Di Bella, et al. 2008. Estrogen deficiency increases osteoclastogenesis up-regulating T cells activity: a key mechanism in osteoporosis. *Bone* Jul;43(1):92–100. Epub 2008 Mar 7. PMID: 18407820.

Pérez, A. V., G. Picotto, A. R. Carpentieri, et al. 2008. Mini-review on regulation of intestinal calcium absorption. Emphasis on molecular mechanisms of transcellular pathway. *Digestion* 77(1):22–34. Epub 2008 Feb 15. PMID: 18277073.

Dick, I. M., A. Devine, J. Beilby, et al. 2005. Effects of endogenous estrogen on renal calcium and phosphate handling in elderly women. *Am J Physiol Endocrinol Metab* Feb;288(2):E430–5. Epub 2004 Oct 5. PMID: 15466921.

Mauras, N., N. E. Vieira, A. L. Yergey. 1997. Estrogen therapy enhances calcium absorption and retention and diminishes bone turnover in young girls with Turner's syndrome: a calcium kinetic study. *Metabolism* Aug;46(8):908–13. PMID: 9258273.

Weaver, C. M. 1994. Age related calcium requirements due to changes in absorption and utilization. *J Nutr* Aug;124(8 Suppl):1418S-1425S. PMID: 8064395.

222. Wright, J. V. and L. Lenard. *Stay Young and Sexy with Bio-Identical Hormone Replacement*, Chapter 6, "Preventing and Reversing Osteoporosis," (Petaluma, CA: Smart Publications), 149.

Prior, J. C. 1990. Progesterone as a bone-trophic hormone. *Endocr Rev* May;11(2):386–98. PMID: 2194787.

Prior, J. C. 2005. Ovarian aging and the perimenopausal transition: the paradox of endogenous ovarian hyperstimulation. *Endocrine* Apr;26(3):297–300. PMID: 16034185.

223. Freeman, S. and L. P. Shulman. 2010. Considerations for the use of progestin-only contraceptives.

J Am Acad Nurse Pract Feb;22(2):81–91. PMID: 20132366.

224. Quinkler, M., K. Kaur, M. Hewison, et al. 2008. Progesterone is extensively metabolized in osteoblasts: implications for progesterone action on bone. *Horm Metab Res* Oct;40(10):679–84. Epub 2008 Jun 6. PMID: 18537080.

Liang, M., E. Y. Liao, X. Xu, et al. 2003. Effects of progesterone and 18-methyl levonorgestrel on osteoblastic cells. *Endocr Res* Nov;29(4):483–501. PMID: 14682477.

Luo, X. H., E. Y. Liao, X. Su. 2002. Progesterone upregulates TGF-b isoforms (b1, b2, and b3) expression in normal human osteoblast-like cells. *Calcif Tissue Int* Oct;71(4):329–34. Epub 2002 Aug 6. PMID: 12154395.

MacNamara, P., C. O'Shaughnessy, P. Manduca, et al. 1995. Progesterone receptors are expressed in human osteoblast-like cell lines and in primary human osteoblast cultures. *Calcif Tissue Int* Dec;57(6):436–41. PMID: 8581876.

Kaunitz, A. M., R. Arias, M. McClung. 2008. Bone density recovery after depot medroxyprogesterone acetate injectable contraception use. *Contraception* Feb;77(2):67–76. PMID: 18226668.

225. Zhang, W. and H. Jia. 2007. Effect and mechanism of cadmium on the progesterone synthesis of ovaries. *Toxicology* Oct 8;239(3):204–12. Epub 2007 Jul 13. PMID: 17719163.

226. Prior, J. C., S. A. Kirkland, L. Joseph, et al. 2001. Oral contraceptive use and bone mineral density in premenopausal women: cross-sectional, population-based data from the Canadian Multicentre Osteoporosis Study. *CMAJ* Oct 16;165(8):1023–9. PMID: 11699697.

227. Hagen, J., N. Gott and D. R. Miller. 2003. Reliability of saliva hormone tests. *J Am Pharm Assoc* Nov-Dec;43(6):724–6. PMID: 14717270.

228. Wright, J. V. and L. Lenard. "Getting the Most Out of BHRT," in *Stay Young and Sexy with Bio-Identical Hormone Replacement*, (Petaluma, CA: Smart Publications), p. 301–308.

229. Rossouw, J. E., G. L. Anderson, R. L. Prentice, et al. 2002. Risks and benefits of estrogen plus progestin in healthy postmenopausal women: principal results From the Women's Health Initiative randomized controlled trial. *JAMA* Jul 17;288(3):321–33. PMID: 12117397.

230. Cauley, J. A., J. Robbins, Z. Chen, et al. 2003. Effects of estrogen plus progestin on risk of fracture and bone mineral density: the Women's Health Initiative randomized trial. *JAMA* Oct 1;290(13):1729–38. PMID: 14519707.

231. Coombs, N. J., K. A. Cronin, R. J. Taylor, et al. 2010. The impact of changes in hormone therapy on breast cancer incidence in the US population. *Cancer Causes Control* Jan;21(1):83–90. Epub 2009 Oct 1. PMID: 19795215.

232. Romieu, I., A. Fabre, A. Fournier, et al. 2010. Postmenopausal hormone therapy and asthma

onset in the E3N cohort. *Thorax* Apr;65(4):292–7. Epub 2010 Feb 8. PMID: 20142267.

Nath, A. and R. Sitruk-Ware. 2009. Different cardiovascular effects of progestins according to structure and activity. *Climacteric* 12 Suppl 1:96–101. PMID: 19811251.

Canonico, M., A. Fournier, L. Carcaillon, et al. 2010. Postmenopausal hormone therapy and risk of idiopathic venous thromboembolism: results from the E3N cohort study. *Arterioscler Thromb Vasc Biol* Feb;30(2):340–5. Epub 2009 Oct 15. PMID: 19834106.

Razavi, P., M. C. Pike, P. L. Horn-Ross, et al. 2010. Long-term postmenopausal hormone therapy and endometrial cancer. *Cancer Epidemiol Biomarkers Prev* Feb;19(2):475–83. Epub 2010 Jan 19. PMID: 20086105.

Shapiro, S. 2007. Recent epidemiological evidence relevant to the clinical management of the menopause. *Climacteric* Oct;10 Suppl 2:2–15. PMID: 17882666.

Pike, M.C., A. H. Wu, D. V. Spicer, et al. 2007. Estrogens, progestins, and risk of breast cancer. *Ernst Schering Found Symp Proc* (1):127–50. PMID: 18540571.

233. Sitruk-Ware, R. 2004. New progestogens: a review of their effects in perimenopausal and postmenopausal women. *Drugs Aging* 21(13):865–83. PMID: 15493951.

234. Puel, C., V. Coxam, M. J. Davicco. 2007. [Mediterranean diet and osteoporosis prevention] *Med Sci* (Paris) Aug-Sep;23(8–9):756–60. PMID: 17875296.

235. Pollan, M. *In Defense of Food* (New York: Penguin Press, 2008), p.1.

236. Dai, Z., Y. Li, L. D. Quarles, T. Song, et al. 2007. Resveratrol enhances proliferation and osteoblastic differentiation in human mesenchymal stem cells via ER-dependent ERK1/2 activation. *Phytomedicine* Dec;14(12):806–14. PMID: 17689939.

Habold, C., I. Momken, A. Ouadi, et al. 2010. Effect of prior treatment with resveratrol on density and structure of rat long bones under tail-suspension. *J Bone Miner Metab* May 11. PMID: 20458604.

Boissy, P., T. L. Andersen, B. M. Abdallah, et al. 2005. Resveratrol inhibits myeloma cell growth, prevents osteoclast formation, and promotes osteoblast differentiation. *Cancer Res* Nov 1;65(21):9943–52. PMID: 16267019.

Zhou, H., L. Shang, X. Li, et al. 2009. Resveratrol augments the canonical Wnt signaling pathway in promoting osteoblastic differentiation of multipotent mesenchymal cells. *Exp Cell Res* Oct 15;315(17):2953–62. Epub 2009 Aug 6. PMID: 19665018.

Liu, Z. P., W. X. Li, B. Yu, et al. 2005. Effects of trans-resveratrol from Polygonum cuspidatum on bone loss using the ovariectomized rat model. *J Med Food Spring* 8(1):14–9. PMID: 15857203.

237. Worthington, V. 1998. Effect of agricultural methods on nutritional quality: a comparison of organic with conventional crops. *Altern Ther Health* Med Jan;4(1):58–69. PMID: 9439021.

238. The Organic Center. Nutrient Decline Linked to the "Dilution" Effect. September 2005 report, http://www.organic-center.org/science.hot.php?action=view&report_id=9 (accessed June 5, 2010).

239. Benbrook, C., X. Zhao, J. Yanes, N. Davies, P. Andrews. "New Evidence Confirms the Nutritional Superiority of Plant-Based Organic Foods," State of Science Review, March 2008, http://www.organic-center.org/science.nutri.php?action=view&report_id=126 (accessed June 5, 2010).

240. Davis, et al. "Changes in USDA Food Composition Data for 43 Garden Crops, 1950 to 1999," *Journal of the American College of Nutrition*, Vol. 23(6): 669–682.

241. Benbrook, C., D. Davis and P. Andrews. "Organic Center Response to the FSA Study," available at http://www.organic-center.org/science.nutri.php?action=view&report_id=157 (accessed June 5, 2010).

242. Worthington, V. 2002. Analyzing data to compare nutrients in conventional versus organic crops. *J*

Altern Complement Med Oct;8(5):529–32. PMID: 12470430.

243. Crinnion, W. J. 2010. Organic foods contain higher levels of certain nutrients, lower levels of pesticides, and may provide health benefits for the consumer. *Altern Med Rev* Apr;15(1):4–12. PMID: 20359265.

Györéné, K. G., A. Varga and A. Lugasi. 2006. [A comparison of chemical composition and nutritional value of organically and conventionally grown plant derived foods] *Orv Hetil* Oct 29;147(43):2081–90. PMID: 17297755.

244. Dahlgren, J. G., H. S. Takhar, C. A. Ruffalo, et al. 2004. Health effects of diazinon on a family. *J Toxicol Clin Toxicol* 42(5):579–91. PMID: 15462149.

Takaro, T. K., L. S. Engel, M. Keifer, et al. 2004. Glycophorin A is a potential biomarker for the mutagenic effects of pesticides. *Int J Occup Environ Health* Jul-Sep;10(3):256–61. PMID: 15473078.

Hrelia, P., C. Fimognari, F. Maffei, et al. 1996. The genetic and non-genetic toxicity of the fungicide Vinclozolin. *Mutagenesis* Sep;11(5):445–53. PMID: 8921505.

Weeks, B. S., S. Lee, P. P. Perez, et al. 2008. Natramune and PureWay-C reduce xenobiotic-induced human T-cell alpha5beta1 integrin-mediated adhesion to fibronectin. *Med Sci Monit* Dec;14(12):BR279–85. PMID: 19043362.

Cho, Y. S., S. Y. Oh, Z. Zhu. 2008. Tyrosine phosphatase SHP-1 in oxidative stress and development of allergic airway inflammation. *Am J Respir Cell Mol Biol* Oct;39(4):412–9. Epub 2008 Apr 25. PMID: 18441283.

Goel, A. and P. Aggarwal. 2007. Pesticide poisoning. *Natl Med J India* Jul-Aug;20(4):182–91. PMID: 18085124.

Arcury, T. A., S. R. Feldman, M. R. Schulz, et al. 2007. Diagnosed skin diseases among migrant farmworkers in North Carolina: prevalence and risk factors. *J Agric Saf Health* Nov;13(4):407–18. PMID: 18075016.

Boutsiouki,P. and G. F. Clough. 2004. Modulation of microvascular function following low-dose exposure to the organophosphorous compound malathion in human skin in vivo. *J Appl Physiol* Sep;97(3):1091–7. PMID: 15333628.

Thrash, B., S. Uthayathas, S. S. Karuppagounder, et al. 2007. Paraquat and maneb induced neurotoxicity. *Proc West Pharmacol* Soc 50:31–42. PMID: 18605226.

245. Sheng, J. P., C. Liu, L. Shen. 2009. [Analysis of some nutrients and minerals in organic and traditional cherry tomato by ICP-OES method] *Guang Pu Xue Yu Guang Pu Fen Xi* Aug;29(8):2244–6. PMID: 19839348.

246. Sheng, J. P., C. Liu, L. Shen. 2009. [Comparative study of minerals and some nutrients in organic celery and traditional celery] *Guang Pu Xue Yu Guang Pu Fen Xi* Jan;29(1):247–9. PMID: 19385250.

247. Raigón, M. D., A. Rodríguez-Burruezo, J. Pro-hens. 2010. Effects of organic and conventional cultivation methods on composition of eggplant fruits. *J Agric Food Chem* Jun 9;58(11):6833–40. PMID: 20443597.

248. Lee, S. H., Y. H. Khang, K. H. Lim, et al. 2010. Clinical risk factors for osteoporotic fracture: a population-based prospective cohort study in Korea. *J Bone Miner Res* Feb;25(2):369–78. PMID: 19594298.

Guadalupe-Grau, A., T. Fuentes, B. Guerra, et al. 2009. Exercise and bone mass in adults. *Sports Med* 39(6):439–68. PMID: 19453205.

249. Donaldson, C. L., S. B. Hulley, J. M. Vogel, et al. 1970. Effect of prolonged bed rest on bone mineral. *Metabolism* Dec;19(12):1071–84. PMID: 4321644.

Krolner, B. and B. Toft. 1983. Vertebral bone loss: an unheeded side effect of therapeutic bed rest. *Clin Sci* (Lond) May;64(5):537–40. PMID: 6831837.

Mazess, R. B. and G. D. Whedon. 1983. Immobilization and bone. *Calcif Tissue Int* May;35(3):265–7. PMID: 6409385.

Ohshima, H. 2006. [Bone loss and bone metabolism in astronauts during long-duration space flight] *Clin Calcium* Jan;16(1):81–5. PMID: 16397355.

250. Kemmler, W., S. von Stengel, K. Engelke, et al. 2010. Exercise effects on bone mineral density, falls, coronary risk factors, and health care costs in older women: the randomized controlled senior

fitness and prevention (SEFIP) study. *Arch Intern Med* Jan 25;170(2):179–85. PMID: 20101013.

Kemmler, W., D. Lauber, J. Weineck, et al. 2004. Benefits of 2 years of intense exercise on bone density, physical fitness, and blood lipids in early postmenopausal osteopenic women: results of the Erlangen Fitness Osteoporosis Prevention Study (EFOPS). *Arch Intern Med* May 24;164(10):1084–91. PMID: 15159265.

Engelke, K., W. Kemmler, D. Lauber, et al. 2006. Exercise maintains bone density at spine and hip EFOPS: a 3-year longitudinal study in early postmenopausal women. *Osteoporos Int* Jan;17(1):133–42. Epub 2005 Aug 12. PMID: 16096715.

Kemmler, W., S. von Stengel, J. Weineck, et al. 2005. Exercise effects on menopausal risk factors of early postmenopausal women: 3-yr Erlangen fitness osteoporosis prevention study results. *Med Sci Sports Exerc* Feb;37(2):194–203. PMID: 15692313.

Angin, E. and Z. Erden. 2009. [The effect of group exercise on postmenopausal osteoporosis and osteopenia] *Acta Orthop Traumatol Turc* Aug-Oct;43(4):343–50. PMID: 19809232.

Asikainen, T. M., K. Kukkonen-Harjula, S. Miilunpalo. 2004. Exercise for health for early postmenopausal women: a systematic review of randomised controlled trials. *Sports Med* 34(11):753–78. PMID: 15456348.

251. Borer, K. T. 2005. Physical activity in the prevention and amelioration of osteoporosis in women: interaction of mechanical, hormonal, and dietary factors. *Sports Med* 35(9):779–830. PMID: 16138787.

252. Iwamoto, J., T. Takeda and S. Ichimura. 2001. Effect of exercise training and detraining on bone mineral density in postmenopausal women with osteoporosis. *J Orthop Sci* 6(2):128–32. PMID: 11484097.

253. Borer, K. T. 2005. Physical activity in the prevention and amelioration of osteoporosis in women: interaction of mechanical, hormonal, and dietary factors. *Sports Med* 35(9):779–830. PMID: 16138787.

254. Hourigan, S. R., J. C. Nitz, S. G. Brauer, et al. 2008. Positive effects of exercise on falls and fracture risk in osteopenic women. *Osteoporos Int* Jul;19(7):1077–86. Epub 2008 Jan 11. PMID: 18188658.

255. Borer, K. T. 2005. Physical activity in the prevention and amelioration of osteoporosis in women: interaction of mechanical, hormonal, and dietary factors. *Sports Med* 35(9):779–830. PMID: 16138787.

256. Specker, B. L. 1996. Evidence for an interaction between calcium intake and physical activity on changes in bone mineral density. *J Bone Miner Res* Oct;11(10):1539–44. PMID: 8889855.

Index